Vegetarian Cooking

for

People with Diabetes

Patricia Le Shane

The Book Publishing Company · Summertown, Tennessee

Cover and interior design by Barbara NcNew
Cover photo by John Guider
Food styling by Mary Anne Fowlkes

On the cover, clockwise from top center: Tropical Fruit Salad, page 137, One-Calorie Herb Dressing, page 79, Basic Free Green Salad, page 70, Tofu-Mushroom Quiche, page 111, Garbanzo-Vegetable Soup, page 89, and Orange Cranberry Muffins, page 66.

ISBN 0-913990-22-1

2 3 4 5 6 7 8 9   © 1994 Patricia Le Shane

The Book Publishing Company
P. O. Box 99
Summertown, TN 38483

Library of Congress Cataloging-in-Publication Data
LeShane, Patricia, 1954-
     Vegetarian cooking for people with diabetes / Patricia LeShane.
          p. cm.
     Includes bibliographical references.
     ISBN 0-913990-22-1
     1. Diabetes--Diet therapy--Recipes. 2. Vegetarian cookery.
I. Title.
RC662.L47 1994
641.5'6314--dc20   94-16298
                                              CIP

Calculations for the nutritional analyses in this book are based on the average number of servings listed with recipes and the average amount of an ingredient if a range is called for. Calculations are rounded up to the nearest gram. If two options for an ingredient are listed, the first one is used. Not included are optional ingredients, serving suggestions, or fat used for frying, unless the amount of fat is specified in the recipe.

Table of Contents

Introduction

When I was first asked if I would consider working on a new revised edition of this book, I didn't realize how much my vegetarianism had evolved and changed. Looking over the recipes, I decided I wanted to update them to reflect more healthful trends in vegetarian diets and the fact that vegetarianism is a healthy choice for people with diabetes.

The most important change was to eliminate all dairy products and eggs from the recipes. Although my reasons for being a vegetarian have always included an awareness of environmental and ethical issues, I have become even more concerned about them. Much damage has been and is continuing to be done to the environment through the use of modern farm factory techniques. These same techniques also involve cruelty and exploitation of animals. There is also the problem of eating the fats contained in meat. In 1990, the largest study ever done on the health effects of consuming animal products was done in China. This study found that the Chinese consume 206 more calories per day than Americans, but that Americans are 25% fatter. This is because over 40% of the calories in the average American diet come from fat, and most of the fat is derived from animal sources. The typical Chinese diet contains less than 15% of calories from fat.

Fat holds higher concentrations of pesticides, hormones, and antibiotics. These chemicals are used because of infestations and infections encouraged by raising crowds of animals in small areas and may be carcinogenic (cancer-causing) to the people who later consume the meat, milk, or eggs from these animals.

These facts, as well as new information about vegetarian, low-fat, high-fiber diets contributed to my desire to update this book. I continue to use basic, healthful ingredients, and the recipes are straight-forward and easy to prepare. I believe in retaining nutrients by shortening cooking time and using raw foods often. The temptation and ease of the fast-food life-style has compromised our health and the health of our planet in recent times. Processed foods, packaged mixes, and micro-wave dinners do not always contain the nutrition we need. They often give us unnecessary doses of preservatives, artificial sweeteners, colors, and other additives. By opening up the world of vegetarian cooking and showing that the diabetic diet can accommodate vegetari-anism very well, I hope this new edition will help people with diabetes and their families live enjoyable, long, healthy lives.

The Two Types of Diabetes

There are two types of diabetes mellitus; insulin-dependent (IDDM) or type I diabetes, (sometimes called juvenile diabetes), and non-insulin-dependent diabetes (NIDDM) or type II diabetes, (sometimes called adult or maturity-onset diabetes).

While the causes of IDDM are not completely understood, both heredity and environment seem to play a part in precipitating its onset. The disease may be caused by a virus or a toxin. Viruses may attack the islet cells of the pancreas and destroy their capability to produce insulin. In some cases, an auto-immune response causes the body to produce anti-insulin antibodies which attack the beta-cells of the pancreas (where insulin is produced). They also attack the insulin molecules.

Without insulin, some cells of the body cannot clear the blood of sugar (glucose) and use it for energy. This causes frequent urination, because glucose stimulates the kidneys to excrete overwhelming amounts of sugar, which the liver would normally conserve. The liver cannot store glucose without insulin. This in turn causes extreme thirst. Weight loss occurs rapidly, because glucose is being washed out of the body, and some of the cells of the body begin to starve. Without insulin, the body burns fat, creating ketones, which cause the blood to become acidic. Lack of insulin also causes increased use of protein for energy. Proteins are converted to glucose in the liver causing further dehydration. Symptoms of IDDM are:

1. Frequent urination
2. Extreme thirst
3. Extreme hunger, as the body tries to feed the starving cells
4. Weight loss, because some cells cannot utilize the food

NIDDM, or type II diabetes, is the most common form of this illness, as many as 85 to 90 percent of the Americans with diabetes are type II. These clients are typically overweight and middle-aged or older. People with NIDDM don't have the extreme symptoms associated with IDDM. The excess blood sugar level is most often discovered during routine medical examinations. The pancreas still makes insulin, but the cells have lost their ability to respond to it. In some cases, the glucose enters the cells but still cannot produce energy. This form of diabetes usually responds well to diet and exercise treatments designed to increase the cells' sensitivity to insulin. The conditions under which type II diabetes can develop are:

1. Inappropriate diet: too much fat, protein, sugar, and simple carbohydrates
2. Obesity (the proportion of fat in the body affects insulin sensitivity)
3. Lack of exercise (inactivity also decreases insulin sensitivity)
4. Vitamin and mineral deficiencies

Diabetes is a serious health problem in this country, consider these facts:

In the United States today, 12 million Americans have diabetes, but only 6 million are aware they have it. Over 600,000 new cases are reported each year. Twice as many black Americans, aged 45 to 65, have diabetes compared to white Americans. Native Americans have the highest rate of NIDDM in the world.

Diabetes is the third leading cause of death by disease.

People with diabetes are twice as likely to have coronary artery disease and three times as likely to suffer a stroke.

Diabetes is also the leading cause of kidney failure.

Infections are more common in people with diabetes.

Another problem is neuropathy, in which the nerves of any part of the body can become sensitive or painful.

Poor circulation, neuropathy, and increased infections can cause long-term foot problems.

Eye problems are another complication of diabetes. Diabetic retinopathy is the most common problem.

As discouraging as all of this may seem, the outlook is much brighter if the person with diabetes can learn to maintain good control of his or her diabetes. With today's increasing knowledge of the importance of diet, exercise, and a better understanding of the disease itself, a person with diabetes can live as long and as comfortably as a person without diabetes.

Being a Vegetarian

There are different ideas about what a vegetarian diet includes. Basically, there are three types. Strict vegetarians or vegans eat no animal foods of any kind. All protein is taken from plant sources. Lacto-vegetarians eat animal protein in the form of milk, cheese, but not meat, fish, poultry, or eggs. Ovo-lacto vegetarians eat animal protein in the form of eggs and dairy products, but not meat, fish, or poultry.

Unfortunately, much of the nonvegetarian public think vegetarians survive on meals of lettuce and broccoli with a few nuts and seeds thrown in for good measure. But this is not true. The plant kingdom contains an enormous variety of foods which can be prepared and combined in a great many ways. In general, vegetarians may be more health conscious than the general public and more concerned with proper nutrition and avoiding processed foods, but this does not mean they are living a deprived existence. The vegetarian diet is an enjoyable diet with much variety.

Throughout history, people have practiced vegetarianism for many reasons. One of the oldest involves a moral question. Some people simply do not believe in killing animals for food. The methods by which animals are raised, slaughtered, and marketed are another reason for them to avoid eating meat.

Other people dislike meat because they think of it as "eating corpses." They feel the sight and smell of dead animals is repulsive, but that a bowl of fruit or a fresh garden vegetable is much more appealing. This feeling for aesthetics is important in defining food choices, not only for vegetarians but anyone. Take, for example, the child who refuses to eat his meal because the "peas are touching the mashed potatoes."

Apart from morality and aesthetics, people may become vegetarians for economic and ecological reasons. Growing vegetables is easier on the land and takes less energy to produce and harvest than animals. More food can be grown in less space. Meat production is more costly. Vegetables and grains that are grown to feed cattle, poultry, and pigs could be fed directly to people instead.

Other people believe that health is the main advantage to being a vegetarian. The mid-1800s marked the beginning of the health food movement in this country. Many reformers were Seventh-Day Adventists and believed that the body should not be fed an unwholesome diet: meat, alcohol, tobacco, or drugs. They, among others, believed that meat consumption led to disease and general bad health and that fruits and vegetables had restorative and cleansing powers. My reason for being a vegetarian is a combination of beliefs. There is the acknowledgment that production of vegetables is better for the world ecologically and economically, as well as a life-long preference for vegetables and the belief that since my diet has consisted mainly of vegetables, I have been, in general, healthier and had more energy than before.

In the first two editions of this book, my recipes were ovo-lacto (that is, contained some dairy and eggs). In this new edition, eggs and dairy have been eliminated. Many new studies have shown that concentrated sources of protein may be worse for a person with diabetes than was previously thought (See Protein, page 12). Also, eating a totally vegan diet is one of the easiest ways to lower your intake of fat a constant problem for someone with diabetes. (See Fat, page 15). Farm animals are often injected with hormones or other drugs to increase their production of milk and eggs. They eat food laced with pesticides and are dosed with insecticides because of the unsanitary conditions caused by overcrowding. All of these substances are concentrated in the bodies of these animals and are passed on to the consumer. Even though vegetable products may also be sprayed, the chemicals do not build up as they do in animals. These days, anything you can do to avoid an extra dose of chemicals may keep you healthier. Many supermarkets now carry organic produce. If you do buy it, you will be encouraging its production and doing your body a favor.

Protein, Carbohydrates & Fats

PROTEIN

Our muscles, skin, hair, nails, eyes, teeth, blood, heart, lungs, brain, and nerves all contain protein. Protein is also involved in metabolism, which is the process that keeps the body growing and maintaining itself. Certain essential substances such as nitrogen, sulfur, and phosphorus, are provided only by protein.

Protein is not stored in the body, so a continuous supply is needed. The cells of the body are constantly breaking down and being replaced every 160 days. Certain organs regenerate even faster. The liver can regenerate damaged tissue almost immediately.

When proteins from food are digested, they are broken down into amino acids, the chemical components that make up protein. If calorie intake is adequate, the amino acids are used for synthesis of body protein. If caloric intake is inadequate, protein intake exceeds what is needed by the body, or all the essential amino acids are not present, protein is converted into glucose or fatty acids and used for energy. There are twenty-two amino acids, but only nine are classified as "essential." The other thirteen are produced by the body if they are not present in the food eaten.

The amino acids are carried by the blood to the liver, from which they are absorbed by the body. They are then recombined to replace worn-out cells, to add to tissues, or to make enzymes, hormones, or other compounds.

The individual's need for protein is determined by body size, age, health, physical activity, and ability of the person to digest and assimilate protein. The quality of protein is also a factor. Meat, fish, poultry, dairy products, and eggs contain all of the essential amino acids. They are "complete" sources. Except for soybeans, vegetable sources are "incomplete." They contain varying amounts of different amino acids. By eating two or more vegetable proteins that make up for each other's deficiencies, a complete protein can be created.

When I wrote the first edition of this book, many nutrition and scientific studies promoted the idea that vegetable proteins which "complemented each other's deficiencies" had to be eaten at he same meal. Frances Moore Lappé, who wrote *Diet For A Small Planet* in 1971 and whose work influenced me, had pioneered this idea. In the 1980s, she revised her work to include new studies on complementary proteins. This research showed that a full protein complement need not be eaten at every meal. However, for the most efficient use of amino acids, they should be eaten within a few hours of each other. A person on a diabetic diet, however, usually eats more than three meals a day. A morning or afternoon snack could be used to compliment the previous meal. For example, the protein in the pasta eaten at lunch could be enhanced by a small cup of lentil soup at snack time. In general, legumes with grains or legumes with nuts or seeds provide full complementation.

This brings us to the question of how much protein we actually need anyway. In recent years, studies have shown that the need is less than previously thought. Many Americans consume 100 or more grams of protein a day. A 150 lb. man actually requires only 35 grams per day. The body uses up a small amount of protein in the production of enzymes and the maintenance of other body proteins. Carbohydrates are the first food burned by the body for energy. While eating too many carbohydrates or fats causes a body to get fat, excess protein cannot be stored. Because of this, it must be broken down and excreted, putting a lot of stress on the body, especially the kidneys. Kidney failure is one of the main complications of diabetes. Diabetes is the main cause of renal failure in the United States. One-fourth of all dialysis patients have diabetes. Eating a vegetarian diet that is high in carbohydrates and low in fats and animal protein is an excellent way to maintain the health of the kidneys.

CARBOHYDRATES

For many people with diabetes, a high complex carbohydrate diet improves the ability to process blood sugar, and in some cases, may stabilize or lower insulin requirements. Most doctors now recommend a diet lower in fat and richer in complex carbohydrates.

Carbohydrates are the main source of energy for the body. They are also needed for the digestion and assimilation of all other foods. Carbohydrates provide instantly available calories for energy and are needed by the liver to break down fats. Protein metabolism is regulated by carbohydrates.

Simple carbohydrates are found in honey, sugar, and fruits. Starches, such as brown rice, potatoes, whole wheat bread, and lentils are complex carbohydrates. All sugars and starches are converted by the digestive system into a simple sugar called glucose. This is the fuel used by the brain, nervous system, muscles, and in body functions.

Carbohydrates provide protein, vitamins, minerals, and are the only source of dietary fiber. For a person with diabetes, foods high in complex carbohydrates are generally low in fat and calories and are satisfying and filling. Hearty meals containing grains, beans, and vegetables fulfill the physical and psychological need for food. Fruits supply nutrients and satisfy a craving for sweetness without an overload of calories and sugar.

FIBER

Fiber is important for people with diabetes. Fiber improves the body's ability to handle blood sugar. A high-fiber diet helps increase the cells' sensitivity to insulin. It also slows down the rise in glucose levels. The fiber content of carbohydrates decreases fat absorption and helps keep blood glucose levels down.

Fiber is an important component in everyone's diet. Found only in plant foods, most fiber is indigestible and supplies no calories, but its bulk helps satisfy the appetite and keeps the digestive system in good condition. Whole grains, beans, fruits, and vegetables are excellent sources of fiber.

Fiber may be soluble or insoluble. Wheat bran is an example of insoluble fiber. It holds water, but doesn't dissolve, and helps food move faster through the intestinal tract. It contributes bulk to waste products and has a laxative effect.

Soluble fiber is found in fruits, vegetables, and beans. This type of fiber slows down the speed at which food goes from the stomach to the intestine.

Both types of fiber help to fill you up without adding unnecessary calories. As you add more fiber to your diet, increase the amount of water you drink to help your body use the fiber effectively and avoid constipation. Don't count on coffee and tea for your liquids, because their diuretic action can deplete your body of fluids

FATS

Eating a low-fat diet is important for the person with diabetes for several reasons. Fat blocks the action of insulin in the blood. Keeping fat intake low is one of the best ways to loose weight and maintain it. A low-fat diet is very important in avoiding some of the serious secondary problems faced by people with diabetes: heart attacks and strokes.

Dietary fats can be placed into two groups: unsaturated and saturated. Unsaturated (including polyunsaturated and monounsaturated) fats are generally liquid at room temperature and are primarily obtained from vegetable and seed oils. Saturated fats are usually solid at room temperature and are mainly from animal sources: lard, butter, and the fat of muscle meats. Coconut and palm oil are saturated vegetable fats.

Hydrogenated fats are polyunsaturated fats that have been changed to solids or partial solids by the addition of hydrogen, making them saturated. These fats are found in processed foods such as shortening margarine, some peanut butters, snack foods, and some candies.

Some fat is essential to the body. A layer of fat under the skin serves as insulation and conserves body heat. Fat also cushions the vital organs and absorbs shock. It is also a component of every cell membrane and is a supply of reserve energy. Fat is needed to house the fat-soluble vitamins and as a source of essential fatty acids. Of these, linoleic acid cannot be made by the body and must be derived from food. Vegetable oils, such as safflower (the highest in linoleic acid), sunflower, corn, soybean, sesame, and peanut oil are sources of this essential acid. Only one tablespoon a day of one of these oils is needed to fill the requirement of an adult for fat. The body can make fat from the two other major nutrients, proteins and carbohydrates. If your diet contains more calories than you need for energy each day, then you "get fat."

Fat is digested more slowly than any other nutrient so its presence delays the return of hunger. However, fats also increase the number of calories that a food provides without contributing much of an increase in nutrients.

The typical American diet contains much more fat than is needed by the body. The greater the saturated fat intake, the greater the chance of the body building up fat deposits and cholesterol in the blood vessels. In general, there is evidence that the populations of countries which consume large amounts of saturated fats (the United States and Europe) have a higher rate of heart disease, obesity, and diabetes. Mediterranean and Asian countries, in general, have a lower rate of these diseases. Their diet contains more vegetable oils and fewer animal products.

Minerals

Minerals are inorganic substances that perform many vital functions in the body. Although not as fragile as vitamins, some are water soluble and can be cooked out of foods, or may be bound by substances in the diet that decrease the body's ability to absorb them.

The minerals which are needed by the body can be placed in two categories. Some are needed in relatively large amounts (macrominerals). These are calcium, phosphorus, magnesium, potassium, sodium chloride, and sulphur. Trace minerals, those needed in very small amounts, are iron, zinc, selenium, manganese, molybdenum, copper, iodine, chromium, fluorine, silicon, chlorine, and cobalt.

MACROMINERALS

Calcium-Calcium aids in muscle contraction and helps maintain the delicate acid-alkaline balance in the body. Heart palpitations can be traced to low calcium levels. Phosphorus and vitamins A, C, and D are needed by the body in order to utilize calcium. Many sources which provide calcium also contain these other substances. Good vegetarian sources of calcium are green vegetables (which are also good suppliers of vitamins A and C), tofu, and cooked beans.

Pregnant women and nursing mothers may need to add about 1 gram (15 grains) of calcium carbonate to their diet each day.

Phosphorus - Phosphorus is used along with calcium in building bones and teeth. It influences protein, carbohydrate, and fat synthesis. It also stimulates muscle contraction, secretion of glandular hormones, nerve impulses, and kidney functioning. Phosphorus is the body's energizer.

A deficiency of phosphorus causes weight and appetite loss, nervous disorder, mental sluggishness, and general fatigue. Deficiencies of this mineral are rare in the United States. Prolonged use of antacids can cause a deficiency and interfere with the calcium-phosphorus balance in the body. Good vegetarian sources of phosphorus are dried beans, peas, whole grains, and vegetables.

Magnesium - Magnesium is important as an enzyme activator in the manufacture of proteins and the release of energy from muscles. It also helps in the conduction of nerve impulses to muscles. A deficiency causes muscular twitching and tremors, irregular heartbeat, insomnia, muscle weakness, cramps, and shaky hands.

Raw, leafy green vegetables, nuts (mainly almonds and cashews), soybeans, seeds, and whole grains are good sources of magnesium.

Potassium- Potassium, together with sodium regulates the heartbeat and muscle contraction, maintains the fluid balance in cells, aids in the transmission of nerve impulses, and releases energy from carbohydrates, proteins and fats.

Potassium stimulates the kidneys to dispose of body wastes. Deficiencies of this mineral cause constipation, nervous disorders, insomnia, irregular heartbeat, and muscle damage.

Good sources of potassium are bananas, citrus fruits tofu, watercress, green peppers chicory, blackstrap molasses, figs, dates, and avocados.

Sodium -Besides working with potassium, sodium works with chlorine in the blood and lymph system. Its main purpose is to make other blood minerals more soluble and prevent them from becoming clogged or deposited in the blood stream.

A sodium deficiency may cause weight loss, stomach and intestinal gas, and muscle shrinkage. Sodium is needed to process amino acids and carbohydrates for digestion. It also helps in the formation of saliva, gastric juices, enzymes, and other intestinal secretions.

Good vegetable sources of sodium are beets, carrots, chard, and dandelion greens.

A deficiency of sodium is less of a problem than too much sodium, usually found in the form of table salt and salt in many of our processed foods. Too much salt has been linked to high blood pressure, heart and kidney disease, and stroke. When a person eats something salty, extra water is drawn from the body in an effort to dilute it. Thirst is stimulated and the kidneys are forced to work hard to excrete the salt. When the body has too much sodium, the kidneys release it into the urine where it is excreted. In some people especially sensitive to sodium the kidneys might not be able to excrete enough of the excess. The excess sodium retains water, and the volume of blood rises. The blood vessels become water-logged and more sensitive to nerve stimulation that causes them to contract. The blood has to pass through narrower channels, and blood pressure increases. The heart rate is speeded up, because there is more blood to pump around the body. Apart from the blood vessels, sodium also increases the amount of water in and around body tissues, which can cause swelling. If this occurs around the heart, heart failure can occur. Swelling in the legs can interfere with blood returning to the heart, and clots may form. Swelling around the brain can cause emotional problems, such as irritability or depression. Sodium also draws water and potassium from the cells of the body. Dried out cells don't function properly and can cause you to feel weak and tired.

For most people all the sodium they need is naturally present in food and water. Exceptions are those people who exercise strenuously for a long time in hot weather. But even for these people, very little salt is needed to regain the proper balance.

Chloride - Chloride works along with sodium to regulate the balance of body fluids and the acid and alkaline levels. It activates the enzyme in saliva and is part of the stomach acid. A deficiency is very rare.

Chloride is a component of table salt, so it is also consumed in excess by many people. Enough chloride to supply the body's needs can be found in the sources which contain natural sodium.

Sulphur - Sulphur is found in amino-acids and is important in the formation of hair, nails, and skin. It helps maintain their smoothness and health. It helps make the blood more resistant to bacterial infections. Sulfur also aids the liver in secreting bile and helps maintain oxygen levels. It works with B-vitamins for metabolism and nerve health.

Deficiencies of this mineral are not known in humans. Enough of this mineral can be obtained through many foods. The best vegetarian sources are wheat germ, dried beans and peas, and peanuts.

TRACE MINERALS

Iron - Iron's main function is in the formation of hemoglobin in the blood and myoglobin in the muscles, which supply oxygen to the cells. Iron also works with other nutrients to help the respiratory system, and is part of some enzymes and proteins.

A shortage of iron can cause anemia, paleness, and poor memory. Good vegetarian sources are dried beans, green leafy vegetables, molasses, and sun-dried raisins.

Zinc - Zinc is an important constituent of insulin. It is also needed to manufacture male hormones. It aids in the storage of glycogen, the utilization of carbohydrates, and the activation of vitamins. Along with phosphorus, zinc aids in the respiration process.

A deficiency can cause slow wound healing and loss of appetite and taste sensation. The best vegetarian sources are whole grains, brewer's yeast, and pumpkin seeds.

Selenium - Selenium is an antioxidant, which prevents the breaking down of fats and other body chemicals. It interacts with vitamin E.

Deficiencies of selenium are not known in humans. Whole grain cereals, broccoli, onions, and garlic are the best vegetable sources.

Manganese - Manganese works with the B-complex vitamins. It helps in building strong bones. Manganese is needed for digestive enzyme function and utilization of food. It also helps the body resist disease and promotes good nerve health.

Deficiencies are not known in humans. Blueberries, green leafy vegetables, peas, beets, and whole grains are the best vegetable sources.

Molybdenum - This mineral is part of some enzymatic processes. Molybdenum deficiency is not known in humans. The best vegetable sources are legumes and cereal grains.

Copper - Copper is needed to convert iron into hemoglobin. It also converts tyrosine, an amino acid, and vitamin C into forms that can be utilized by the body. A deficiency of copper causes skin sores to develop and not heal, general weakness, and poor respiration. Vegetable sources are almonds, dried beans, dried peas, whole wheat, and prunes.

Iodine - Iodine stimulates the thyroid gland to make the thyroxine hormone, essential to the function of the gland. It also is needed to utilize fat. A deficiency causes slow mental reaction, rapid pulse, heart palpitation, tremor, nervousness, irritability, restlessness, and dry hair. The best vegetable sources are vegetables grown in iodine-rich soil, kelp, other sea vegetables, and onions.

Chromium - Chromium is necessary for the metabolism of glucose. A deficiency may possibly lead to adult-onset diabetes. Whole grains, dried beans, peanuts, and brewer's yeast are the best sources.

Fluoride - This mineral helps to prevent tooth decay and strengthen tooth enamel, but too much can have the opposite effect. Fluoridated water and vegetable foods grown with fluoridated water are the best sources.

Silicon - Silicon is needed for strong bones and teeth. It is found in the cells of the hair, muscles, nails, and connective tissues. A deficiency can cause fatigue, glazed and dull eyes, and puffy skin.

The best vegetable sources are buckwheat products, mushrooms, carrots, and tomatoes.

Cobalt - Cobalt is a component of vitamin B12. Its sources are mainly of animal origin, but some is found in sea vegetables.

Vitamins

Vitamins are absolutely essential for all bodily processes but are needed only in small amounts. They work with enzymes to process fats, carbohydrates, proteins, and minerals. They help form blood cells, hormones, genetic material, and certain body chemicals. Because vitamins have so many roles, a deficiency of one may affect more than one body function. The lack of different vitamins may produce similar deficiency symptoms.

There are two categories of vitamins: fat-soluble and water-soluble. Fat-soluble vitamins are stored in body fat, so it is not essential to consume them daily. Water-soluble vitamins are not stored in the body and must be supplied daily, because they are constantly being excreted through urine and perspiration.

Vitamin A - This is a fat-soluble vitamin that is stored mainly in the liver. The body requires adequate protein in order to utilize this vitamin. The main functions of vitamin A are the maintenance of healthy skin, hair, and mucous membranes, to aid in night vision the ability, and to promote and maintain the development of bones and teeth.

Lack of vitamin A can make it difficult to withstand viral infections. The hair and skin can become dry and brittle and the eyes red and itchy.

Vitamin A is easily oxidized (a reaction with oxygen causing spoilage) and needs vitamin E to help prevent this. This vitamin is easily destroyed by light, prolonged heat, and rancidity of fats. It is stable in short cooking times. Carrots and dark green vegetables should be steamed lightly to obtain the optimum amount of vitamin A.

The best vegetarian sources of vitamin A are yellow, orange, and dark green vegetables.

Vitamin B Complex - B-vitamins are water soluble and are needed for all the living cells to carry out their metabolic processes. The B-complex vitamins are dependent on one another and an inadequate intake of one may affect the utilization of the others. White rice, flour, and sugar have had all the B-vitamins refined out of them. B-vitamins are also destroyed by intense heat, excessive cooking, and light. Baking soda and baking powder also destroy some vitamin B.

B-vitamins are responsible for the health of the digestive tract, the skin, mouth, tongue, eyes, nerves, arteries, and liver, as well as proper metabolism. Deficiencies cause skin disorders, mental confusion, irritability, muscular weakness and cramps, anemia, smooth tongue, mouth swelling, fatigue, difficulty sleeping, tingling sensations in the hands and feet, and depression.

Vitamin B_{12} is produced only by microbes and naturally occurs only in animal products. Vegetarians who do not use eggs or dairy products need to supplement vitamin B_{12}. Some brands of texturized vegetable protein, tofu, nutritional yeast, spirulina, miso, and tempeh contain added B_{12}. Extra B_{12} is stored mainly in the liver. A shortage of this essential vitamin can cause severe damage to the nervous system.

Vitamin C - Vitamin C is water soluble and aids in the good health of the body by protecting against colds and building resistance to fatigue and stress. This vitamin is concentrated in the white blood cells, which fight infections. Vitamin C brings hydrogen into the body and helps in metabolism. It also helps in absorption of iron, in healing wounds, and nurturing bones, skin, teeth, and blood vessels. Vitamin C is also a good natural laxative because it dilutes bile which breaks down fat. It is advisable for people who do prolonged hard physical work, consume chemically fertilized food, or are exposed to air pollution, cigarette smoke, mental stress, or infections, to increase their daily vitamin C intake.

A deficiency is marked by weakness, aches, bruising, internal hemorrhaging, bleeding gums, swelling joints, and shortness of breath.

The best sources are citrus fruit juices: orange, grapefruit, lemon, lime, and grape. The vegetarian foods richest in vitamin C are tomatoes, strawberries, melons, green peppers, potatoes, dark green vegetables, and alfalfa.

Vitamin C is water soluble and cannot be stored in the body. It must be ingested daily. It is sensitive to heat, so vitamin C foods are best eaten raw, or in the case of potatoes, not overcooked. Potatoes should be steamed to avoid contact with water which leaches out the vitamin content.

Vitamin D - Vitamin D is a fat-soluble vitamin which is used with calcium in the formation of bones and teeth. It is necessary for the absorption of calcium and phosphorus. When skin is exposed to the sun, oils in the skin react with the sunlight and synthesize vitamin D.

A prolonged deficiency will cause rickets, a disease which affects children by stunting bone growth and causing malformed teeth and a protruding abdomen. In adults, osteomalacia may result. This is a softening of the bones which can lead to fractures, muscle spasms, and twitching.

Sunlight is the most efficient source of this vitamin.

Vitamin E - This vitamin's main function is to prevent fatty acids from reacting with oxygen and to slow deterioration of the cells. It acts as a natural "preservative." It helps to protect vitamin A, and aids in the formation of red blood cells, muscles, and other tissues. It is a fat-soluble vitamin and is stored in the body. The refining of wheat into white bread, and the heating and hydrogenation of vegetable oil destroys vitamin E. It is possible that the decrease of vitamin E in our bodies since these practices began may be a contributing factor in the increase in heart disease and heart attacks that we are experiencing today. Vitamin E is depleted from the body when called upon to prevent oxidation of fats.

Depletion of vitamin E may cause muscular weakness, oxidized fat deposits, and interference with hormone production.

The best sources for vitamin E are vegetable oil, wheat germ, whole grain cereals, bread, dried beans, and green leafy vegetables.

Vitamin K - Vitamin K is a fat-soluble vitamin and needs the presence of bile, which is made by the liver, to be absorbed. It is stable in heat, but is destroyed by light. The main function of this vitamin is to stimulate the production of prothrombin in the blood by the liver. A deficiency will cause blood clotting to take place too slowly.

Enough vitamin K is present in the average diet. It can also be made by the intestines. Impaired fat absorption, liver disease, the prolonged use of antibiotics or sulphur drugs, or an extremely poor diet are the rare causes of deficiency.

The best vegetarian sources of this vitamin are alfalfa, kale, spinach, and cabbage.

Vegetarian Foods

The vegetarian diet offers a wonderful variety of foods. If you are just becoming a vegetarian, look at this as a chance to explore a whole new world of tastes and aromas. Here are some tips to help you get started.

GRAINS AND FLOURS

In parts of the world other than the United States, grains provide people with most of their protein. Rice, millet, cracked wheat, barley, buckwheat, and corn are the most widely used, mainly in an unrefined state. In North America and much of Europe, however, rice and wheat, the most commonly used grains, are refined into white rice and white flour. The refining process removes the hull of the grain, the bran, and the germ. Refining also removes most of the protein, fiber, calcium, phosphorus, iron, vitamin E, and the B vitamins. In the case of white rice, the grain is then polished, coated with a mixture of alcohol and zein (a protein derivative from corn), then treated with calcium and iron salts, dipped into the mix again, and treated with synthetic vitamins, this enrichment does not put back all the nutrients lost in the refining process.

Once you start using brown rice, barley, oats, wheat, millet, and corn, you will discover there is more variety in the dishes you prepare with no extra work. When you cook grains, the measurement of water to grain does not need to be exact. Usually a dry grain will need a pot big enough to allow it to triple in volume. Two cups of water to one cup of grain is the basic proportion. (See chart for cooking times on page 44.)

Check bread labels for the words "whole wheat flour." "Wheat" flour means the same as "white" flour in the commercial bread baking world. According to the USDA federal standard, if a bread is said to be "whole wheat," it must be 100% whole wheat.

Commercially baked bread may also contain more than a hundred food and chemical additives. Specialty breads, like rye, pumpernickel, corn, or other combinations may contain more white flour than whole flours from which they were traditionally made. For example, pumpernickel, which should be made of a combination of rye and whole wheat flours, may be mainly white flour with only 2% rye flour and caramel coloring and molasses added to give the appearance of pumpernickel.

If you cannot find a suitable whole wheat bread, buy flour and enjoy the satisfaction of baking your own. Whole wheat flour can be found in any supermarket. Keep it in the refrigerator or in a very cool place to avoid rancidity.

Flour can be made from any grain. Whole wheat flour and cornmeal can be found in supermarkets, but buckwheat or rice flours are harder to come by. If you really get involved in experimenting with various flours, home grain mills can be purchased through magazine ads (in magazines like *Country Journal, Organic Gardening, Yankee, Sunset* or other cooking and gardening publications) or possibly at your local appliance store.

One flour you can make in a regular blender is oat flour. Pour 1 cup of rolled oats into the blender or food processor, and grind until it is reduced to a powder. Oat flour absorbs water and can create a heavy bread if used alone, but gives a nice variation in taste when it is mixed with whole wheat flour. It also can be used to make a more nutritious thickener than cornstarch.

READY-TO-EAT CEREALS & CRACKERS

My favorite cold cereal is simply cold cooked rice, millet, bulgur, or barley. If you like a crunchy breakfast but don't know which ready-to-eat cereal is best as far as taste and nutrition, try using plain wheat germ with fruit and soy yogurt. It offers excellent nutrition with good taste, but no sugar, preservatives, or additives. Mix wheat germ with rolled oats, nuts, or seeds for variety. Watch out for packaged granola cereals. Even though they may be "all natural," they may be very high in sugar and fat. Wheat flakes, rye flakes, and muesli cereals are worth trying, as are any cold cereals made of unprocessed oats, millet, corn, wheat germ, seeds, and dried fruit. Avoid cereals with BHT and BHA.

The best rule for buying crackers is the simpler the better. Many crackers are made from only water and whole wheat flour. Try to use crackers without white flour, sugars, artificial color and flavor, sodium propionate, disodium acetate, or BHA and BHT. Often, the best crackers may not be in the regular cookie/cracker section, but in the gourmet or dietetic section.

LEGUMES

Along with grains, legumes are the primary source of protein for the vegetarian. Some of the legumes I have listed are more common than others, but all of them are well worth trying.

Black beans are best in soups. They become very soft in cooking and create a hearty, thick soup.

Black-eyed peas are small and oval shaped. They are white in color with one black "eye," and are popular in southern and soul food cookery.

Garbanzo beans seem to go well with every grain. They may be used in main dishes, soups, sandwiches, and salads. They are a tan, round-shaped bean, and take a longer time to cook than most beans except soy.

Great northern beans and navy beans are the beans most of us have eaten as "baked beans." They are also good in soups.

Kidney beans and pinto beans are often used interchangeably. Kidney beans are red and kidney shaped. Pintos are beige with dark speckles. They go well with all grains and are good in soups and casseroles.

Lentils can be red, green, or brown in color. They are tiny and look like split peas. They cook in only 30-40 minutes and are excellent in soups and casseroles.

Lima beans are a flat, white bean. You may be more familiar with frozen, green lima beans. Dried lima beans are good for soups and casseroles.

Peanuts are officially legumes, but see them in the "Nut and Seeds" section.

Split peas come in green and yellow. The yellow have a slightly less pronounced flavor. Both varieties are cooked in the same way. Soup is the traditional use for split peas, but they can be served with a grain or in casseroles.

Soybeans and their products deserve a whole cookbook for themselves. They are the only food in the vegetable kingdom, apart from nutritional yeast, that contains all the essential amino acids. Whole, cooked soybeans can be used in many ways: soups, casseroles, salads, or pureed into a sandwich spread. Soybeans, like all other beans, must be cooked until they are completely soft.

Soy grits are toasted pieces of the soybean. They can be added to casseroles or bread to give it a chopped nut effect but with fewer calories and less fat.

Tofu, a versatile soybean product, is a solid white cake of bean curd, made in a way that is similar to the cheese-making process. Tofu has a smooth texture and mild flavor which blends well with any food. It needs no cooking which makes it good for fast meals, salads, and sandwiches. Because soybeans are high in oil, the fat content of regular tofu is over 40%. Because the total number of calories in an average serving is very low, this doesn't amount to a great deal of fat. However, for anyone who eats a lot of tofu and watches fat grams carefully, there are some new types of tofu currently available. There is reduced-fat tofu which is 32% less fat than regular tofu. It is made by removing the hulls of the beans before they are processed. There is also a brand new product called low-fat tofu that is made from regular tofu, soy isolate (the pure protein extracted form the bean), and fermented cornstarch. Low-fat tofu is only 1% fat.

Tempeh is a high-protein food made from soybeans or grains through a natural culturing process. It contains more riboflavin, niacin, and B6 than regular soybeans. It is low in calories and cholesterol-free. The flavor of tempeh depends on what bean, grain and bean, or nut combination it is made from. Most of the tempeh in this country is made from soybeans and is available at health food stores. Tempeh is the most digestible form of soybeans. Keep tempeh refrigerated and steam it for 10 minutes before using. Tempeh can be diced or grated to add protein, vitamins, and minerals to salads, sandwiches, soups, and casseroles. Marinating in herbs, spices, or tamari can vary the flavor of tempeh. You can combine it with grains and vegetables.

Soy flour is a heavy flour which can add complete protein to your home baked foods. It should never be eaten raw. Use it only in thoroughly cooked dishes or baked goods. Soy flour has a strong, nutty taste. Use ¼ cup to each cup of whole wheat flour.

Texturized vegetable protein is made from defatted soy flour. The soy flour has had the oil extracted from it and what remains is mostly protein and carbohydrate. The defatted soy flour is cooked under pressure and extruded through holes, then cut into pieces of various sizes. This dry, precooked food can then be rehydrated and made into many dishes. If you cannot find texturized vegetable protein in your local market, you can get it from The Mail Order Catalog, P. O. Box 180, Summertown, TN 38483, phone 1-800-695-2241.

Tamari is a type of soy sauce. It is naturally aged and contains no chemical colorings, as many soy sauces do. However, it is high in sodium and should be used sparingly.

Most legumes are available in supermarkets. Soybean products, such as tofu and tempeh are becoming more common in many markets. In some areas, a natural foods store or co-op may be the best place to find them.

NUTS AND SEEDS

Nuts and seeds are as rich in protein as legumes. They are more filling and are higher in calories and fat. While nuts and seeds can add flavor and texture to many dishes, they can also greatly increase the percentage of fat in a meal (dried sunflower seeds are 72% fat). So use them sparingly.

Seeds have more usable protein than nuts. Sunflower seeds are the best. They supply good quality protein and are an important source of Vitamin B_6. They are also lower in calories per gram of usable protein than sesame seeds or nuts.

Nuts are sold shelled and unshelled, except for cashews which are never in a shell. Unshelled nuts have the advantage of the shell as a guard against nutritional loss and chemical contamination. Unshelled nuts are treated with lye and gas to soften and loosen them from the shell. Shells are usually bleached and may be colored or waxed. Use pistachios that haven't been dyed red. Inspect unshelled nuts to be sure they have no mold and a minimum of shell damage.

Nuts in the shell are unroasted, except for peanuts. Shelled nuts, however, may be raw or roasted and whole or in pieces. Almonds are blanched in a hot-water bath to remove the outer skin, a process done for cosmetic reasons only. Unblanched almonds are also available and contain more nutrients.

Avoid buying unshelled nuts that have been roasted in oil and salt. They have too much additional fat roasted into them. Look for unsalted, dry roasted nuts.

Nuts and seeds must be protected from heat, air, and moisture. They should be stored shelled or unshelled in a covered container in a cool place. In hot weather, keep them in the refrigerator.

Nuts and seeds are a good addition to any vegetarian meal. Use them in main dishes, breakfast cereals, pancakes, baked products, salads, sandwiches, vegetable stir-fry dishes, and many other ways. Any nuts or seeds can be ground into nut butter, similar to peanut butter. If you want to do this at home, be sure to keep track of the amount of nuts and the amount of oil you use. Basically, 2 cups of nuts ground into a powder with ¼ cup of safflower oil, added slowly, is a good mixture. One tablespoon of most nut butters can be counted the same as peanut butter (1 high-fat meat exchange or 1 lean meat exchange plus 1 fat exchange).

Buy peanut butter made only from peanuts. Avoid brands that contain sugars, hydrogenated shortening, and salt. You may not be able to get salt-free brands in a supermarket, but most natural food stores have them. It is better to add a small amount of salt yourself, if you are trying to use less, but haven't gotten away from it completely.

VEGETABLES

Grains, legumes, nuts, and seeds are important sources of protein, minerals, vitamin B complex, and vitamin E. Vegetables are needed to round out vitamin and mineral requirements. Except for vitamin D, every vegetable is strong in one or more of the essential vitamins and minerals. A good variety of vegetables will cover all the nutrients. The nutritional value of vegetables varies with the kind of vegetable, the season of harvesting, soil, storage, and preparation. In general, certain vegetables can be counted on for certain nutrients. All yellow, orange, and dark green vegetables are rich in vitamin A. Green leafy vegetables also supply vitamin C, iron, riboflavin, and calcium. When fresh, most vegetables are a reliable source of vitamin C, especially when eaten raw.

Sprouts are easy to grow and are a good source of protein, vitamin C, and trace minerals. By growing sprouts, you can always have a fresh vegetable to add to soups, sandwiches, and salads. See page 74 for directions for growing them.

In most cases, vegetables are at their best nutritionally if they are eaten soon after harvesting. Of course, this isn't always possible. Nutritional losses occur from chemical changes taking place within the plant. These changes can be accelerated by heat or slowed down by cold.

Packaged frozen vegetables go from the field to the freezing and packing plant. They may be frozen immediately, or they may lose vitamins for a few days before they are processed. The consumer has no way of knowing. In addition, these vegetables may be sprayed with chemicals to avoid spoilage while they are waiting to be frozen. Before they are frozen, they are blanched with hot water to destroy certain enzymes which cause spoilage during storage. This process does destroy some vitamin C and other vitamins. When frozen vegetables arrive at the super market, there is no way to know how long they have been in the freezer case. Even when they are taken home, they may not be used for another week or more. Although freezing slows down the nutritional loss, the older the vegetables become, the greater the loss. If the vegetables have become partially defrosted through mishandling at any point in the process, further spoilage occurs.

With all those chances for nutritional loss, freezing is still better than canning. The heat involved in canning changes the color, flavor, and texture of the vegetables or fruit. It also destroys much of the vitamin content. Many nutrients are lost in the water in which the vegetables are canned. Canned vegetables are also subjected to the addition of acids to ensure the retardation of bacterial growth. Acids (usually baking soda) destroy B vitamins. Salt, sugar, artificial coloring and flavoring, and other additives may also be used in processing.

Fresh vegetables are best. Still, it may not be known how fresh they are or if they have been sprayed. Locally grown produce is your best bet. Try to fit those into your meals when they are available. If you are lucky enough to live in a section of the country where there is always some variety of vegetable in season, use what is fresh. If you live in the north, have plenty of squash, green beans, tomatoes, etc., all summer and forget frozen vegetables until the fresh ones in the markets begin to look like they've been on a long, slow train. Be sure to wash all fresh vegetables well. Do not soak them, but scrub them in cold, soapy water. Soaps can remove some chemicals that plain water cannot. Rinse them well. Select vegetables that look fresh and have no bruises. Handle them carefully and buy only what you need. Plan to eat them within one or two days. Root vegetables such as potatoes, carrots, parsnips, onions, turnips, can be kept longer, but they will also suffer some nutritional loss.

Vegetables should be peeled only when the skin is unpalatable, such as turnips, rutabagas, or the tough stem ends of broccoli. Cook yams, squash, and potatoes in their skins. Peel them when cooked or eat the peel too (yes, even butternut or acorn squash).

Steaming is my favorite method for cooking vegetables, because it is easy, fast, and there is no contact with water. This minimizes the loss of nutrients. Steaming also helps to preserve the bright color of the vegetables. Broccoli retains its bright green and winter squash its bright orange. Boiling creates dull, soggy, tasteless food. Steaming also retains flavor, which helps reduce the need for salt.

Pressure cooking is also an excellent method. Timing must be accurate or the vegetables can quickly become overcooked. The greatest percentage of vitamins is retained using this method.

Cooking times for steaming or pressure cooking vary from vegetable to vegetable. Also, the same vegetable can vary, one bunch of broccoli may be tougher than another, or the green beans bought this shopping trip may be larger than last week's. Experiment and cook until the vegetable is just tender, not mushy. When steaming vegetables, you will find that if you turn off the heat when they are half done, they will keep cooking if kept tightly covered. Frozen vegetables need little more than to be heated thoroughly by the steam, because they have already been blanched.

The best tips to remember for vegetables are to buy fresh, seasonal vegetables first, fresh, good-looking vegetables that are in their peak season wherever they came from second, frozen vegetables third, and canned vegetables least often. Organically grown vegetables have had no chemicals used in their production.

FRUITS

Fruit provides the body with natural sugar to satisfy the craving for sweets. Adding fruit to your daily diet also helps fill vitamin and mineral requirements. Most fruits contain varying amounts of vitamins A and C, potassium, some calcium, and iron.

As with vegetables, the best fruit you can get is in season and grown locally. Fruits are usually grown in chemically fertilized soil. Fruit trees and bushes are sprayed with herbicides and pesticides, unless they are organic. Some fruits have a protective outer layer which is never eaten. The edible part is protected from surface spraying. Examples include pineapples, bananas, and melons; apples, pears, peaches, and other fruits have no such protection. All fruits and vegetables should be scrubbed thoroughly before eating. Grapes, in particular, are heavily sprayed and need to be thoroughly washed.

Fruits are often waxed or colored to make them look more appealing and fresh. Oranges growing on trees are not bright orange and lemons are not such a bright yellow. Grating these rinds into your cooking ingredients may add some dangerous dyes into your food.

Waxed apples, pears, or any extremely shiny fruit should be peeled. Many vitamins reside in the peel, but the wax is almost impossible to remove.

Unfortunately, many fruits are picked when immature and never ripen sufficiently. They may become dried out and tasteless, instead of juicy and sweet.

Pick fruit that has good color naturally, such as firm red or green apples with no bruises, preferably unwaxed. Bananas should be partially green and have few surface bruises. Wait until their jackets are a mellow yellow with a few brown speckles before eating; this is the peak of their ripeness. When buying berries, do not buy light colored ones (immature), or ones that look overripe; they should be plump and firm. When buying citrus, pick fruits that feel heavy for their size. Thin-skinned citrus are juicier. Avoid ones that yield to pressure (true of any fruit). Buy uncolored citrus if it is available. Peaches, nectarines, and plums should be rich in color. Melons are often difficult fruits to judge for ripeness. Look for ones with even color and with a slight softening at the blossom end.

Fruits should be stored in the refrigerator unless they need a day or two to ripen. Bananas can be refrigerated when ripe. The outer peel will turn dark brown, but the banana itself will remain firm.

Fortunately, fruits have a higher natural acid content than vegetables, and so lose fewer vitamins in the canning process. The peeling, cutting, and heating of the canning process does decrease some of the nutrients, and as with vegetables, most of these nutrients are lost if the canning water is thrown out.

Fruits are rich in natural sugars, but manufacturers add sugar to canned fruits to maintain the texture and as a preservative. It is possible to buy only lightly sweetened fruit or fruit preserved in its own juice. The label must state if sugar is added, *so read the label.*

Frozen fruits may also have sugar added, particularly frozen berries. They may also have added colorings, salt, or acids. It is best to choose fresh seasonal fruits and avoid canned or frozen ones.

People with diabetes are often warned to stay away from dried fruit because they are a concentrated source of sugar. It is true that only 3 prunes, 1½ figs, or 2 tablespoons of raisins equal one fruit exchange. Yet, it is possible to enjoy these fruits in small amounts because their flavor is also concentrated. They can add a lot of taste to a dish of oatmeal or a cup of soy yogurt. Use them in the amounts suggested for one serving, and they will give you a naturally sweet treat with all the iron and nutrients of fresh fruit. The drying process retains the vitamins and minerals.

If possible, get sun-dried and not artificially dehydrated fruit. This latter method uses sulphur dioxide, which is always stated on the label. Some sun-dried fruits contain sulphur too. Other ingredients to avoid are added sugar, corn syrup, honey, and preservatives.

MAYONNAISE, OIL AND SALAD DRESSINGS

Bottled salad dressings have an amazingly long list of ingredients, considering these foods should be a simple blend of oil, vinegar, herbs, and spices. They may also contain salt, sugar, MSG, stabilizers, emulsifiers, preservatives, coloring, and starches. Many brands use strong, cheap white vinegar and cottonseed oil, pressed from the same seeds that are harvested with cotton. Since cotton's main use is not as a food crop, it is heavily sprayed, compromising the quality of the seed oil. It is safer to make your own dressings (see recipes).

Mayonnaise can contain many undesirable ingredients, such as sugars, starches, and preservatives. I recommend using tofu mayonnaise, because no egg yolks are used. There are currently vegetarian alternatives available that are tasty and lower in fat.

When buying oil, you will find that the most common product is "pure vegetable oil." This is no assurance of purity. Fortunately, the type of oil is identified on the label. Again, look for brands that don't contain cottonseed oil. Avoid oils with preservatives such as BHA, BHT, and polysorbate 80.

Corn, canola, safflower, peanut, and soybean oils are excellent sources of polyunsaturated fat. Try to get these in brands without additives. Olive oil is the only oil that is always unrefined and contains no additives. It is cold-pressed, which means it is removed from the plant by pressing, instead of using heat or solvents which destroy vitamin E, a natural antioxidant. Refined oils can become rancid. Manufacturers add chemicals to slow this process. However, if you buy refined, unpreserved oils and use them within a month or two, no rancidity should occur if they are kept in the refrigerator.

Ultimately, the best recommendation for all of these fats is to use them sparingly.

HONEY AND MOLASSES

In my recipes, I occasionally use blackstrap molasses or honey in small amounts. I feel that these are better than using chemical sugar substitutes or white sugar. When sugarcane goes through processing to yield white sugar, the residue is blackstrap molasses. It contains all the nutrients of the original sugar cane, which are B vitamins, calcium, phosphorus, and iron. Blackstrap molasses has a strong, almost bitter taste; very little is needed in a recipe. Unsulphured molasses also contains the same nutrients as blackstrap, but has a mellower taste. It is not a by-product of sugar refining but is manufactured for the molasses itself.

Honey, the nectar of flowers which is converted to a rich syrup by bees, is another sugar substitute that can be used in small amounts. You may prefer to buy unfiltered, raw honey. This honey has not been subjected to heat and so contains traces of nutrients and enzymes. Because honey may contain botulism spores, health professionals warn against feeding it to infants under one year of age, because they may be especially sensitive to those spores. Raw honey and unsulphured molasses can be found in supermarkets. Blackstrap molasses may be found in natural food stores or co-ops.

TOMATO SAUCE

Buy only the brands of tomato sauce that do not contain artificial color, artificial flavor, preservatives, starchy thickeners, corn syrup, sugar, or salt. It is better to add a little salt yourself, if you must. In my recipes, I use only a small amount of tomato sauce. I prefer to use vegetables with the sauce to create a more interesting flavor. Tomato sauce is a good, low-fat alternative to cream or cheese sauces, but if you're not careful, tomato sauce calories can add up quickly.

NUTRITIONAL AND BREWER'S YEAST

Nutritional yeast (saccharomyces cerevisiae) grown in a molasses solution has a delicious flavor somewhat like cheese. It provides B vitamins and quality protein. Children like it sprinkled on pasta, rice, other grains, beans, popcorn, and vegetables. It is easily digestible and contains all the essential amino acids. Its riboflavin content gives it a yellow color. Try using nutritional yeast in casseroles, sprinkled on cereals, added to soups and gravies, or in blended drinks.

Nutritional yeast comes in both flakes and powder and is available at health food stores. If you cannot find nutritional yeast in your local market, you can get it from The Mail Order Catalog, P. O. Box 180, Summertown, TN 38483, phone 1-800-695-2241. No more than 3 teaspoons of powder or 4 teaspoons of flakes should be eaten per person per day. Check the label of the yeast you buy to see if it has vitamin B_{12}. This important vitamin is the one most likely to be deficient in a total vegetarian diet. The inclusion of good tasting nutritional yeast daily will help supply B_{12}.

Brewer's yeast is a by-product of the beer-making process. It does not have the same taste as nutritional yeast but is still an excellent source of the B-vitamin complex and a source of complete protein. It can be found in any natural food store or co-op, or in many supermarkets. Yeast is also available in pill form as a food supplement.

Yeast is also a source of the trace mineral chromium, which has been studied as a possible aid in the treatment of adult-onset diabetes. Chromium seems to enhance the insulin production of the pancreas. It is believed that a deficiency of this mineral may be a factor in the development of diabetes.

KELP

Kelp is the general name for various large, brown sea vegetables which are rich in iodine and other minerals. It is a good addition to a low-salt diet, because it provides iodine without the sodium. It is available in tablets or powder in natural food stores and some drug stores. It is preferable to use the powder, because the tablets, by law, can contain only 0.15 milligrams of iodine. Try using kelp by adding it to any casserole, salad dressing, or soup.

COFFEE AND TEA

There are many brands and flavors of herbal teas on the market today. Take a break from regular coffee and tea, and experiment with a wide variety of caffeine-free teas. You may find that they soothe your nerves after a long day much better than black teas or coffee.

The caffeine in tea and coffee can have a variety of effects on the body. It is a stimulant, which helps wake you up in the morning or pick you up late in the day. It has a direct, stimulating effect on the parts of the brain which affect mental processes, heart rate, respiration, and muscle coordination. It can raise the basal metabolic rate and so increase the number of calories burned, but it also ignites the release of insulin, causing blood sugar to drop.

The positive effect of caffeine is that it stimulates blood flow to the heart by dilating the coronary arteries. It also constricts the blood vessels which go to the brain and is included in some headache remedies, since dilated blood vessels contribute to headaches.

There are more potential hazards than good points about caffeine, however. Caffeine is an addictive substance, and for all it can do to relieve headaches, it can addict you to the remedy. Excessive caffeine can produce an abnormally fast heart beat and also increase blood pressure. It is also linked to ulcers and other digestive problems. Heartburn is often the result of too much coffee or tea. Anxiety and muscular jitters are other problems caused by too much caffeine.

Along with caffeine, the tannic acid in tea, the dyes used in the black or orange pekoe leaves, and the chemicals in tea bags are also health concerns. Try to reduce or eliminate coffee and tea in your diet. If you still wish to drink it, try brewing the tea for a shorter time and don't let perked coffee stand with the coffee grounds. Reduce your consumption to two or three cups a day. Remember to count the extra calories if you use sweeteners.

LEAVENING AGENTS

Baking soda, baking powder, and yeast are leavening agents. Baking soda works by releasing carbon dioxide when it is mixed with a liquid. Baking powder is made of baking soda, an acid salt, which produces a more controlled leavening action, and a starch, which prevents the powder from caking. Yeast works by giving off carbon dioxide as the result of fermentation. Fermentation begins when the yeast is mixed with a warm liquid.

Yeast is the best leavening agent. It contains B vitamins and destroys none of the nutrients in the baked product. Unfortunately, baking soda and baking powder, which may seem the easiest to use, affect the nutrient thiamine in the flour. Some of the B vitamins are destroyed. There is also concern that aluminum-based baking powders may have negative health effects. Use baking powder that does not contain aluminum, but uses tartar or phosphate in the ingredients. The use of whole wheat flour and wheat germ, with their higher amounts of B vitamins, is especially important if baking powders are used.

Diet and Shopping Tips

1. Take advantage of the "free" foods (no calories) allowed in the diabetic diet. Just a few raw vegetables, such as cucumbers and celery, eaten at lunch and dinner can help satisfy your appetite while adding vitamins, minerals, enzymes, and fiber to your diet.

2. Skip the oil on your salad, and save on fat calories by using only vinegar or lemon juice. Try wine vinegar, cider vinegar, and herb vinegars.

3. Fats can be reduced or eliminated by using non-stick cookware. The following recipes will indicate where these utensils have been used and if there is a significant difference in fats.

4. Experiment with various herbs to help eliminate your salt craving. Take the salt shaker off of the table, and replace it with a mixture of your favorite herbs, or try some of the commercial mixes that are available. See the herb mix in the recipe section page 138.

5. Try drinking herbal teas. There is a large selection to choose from. Add a pinch of cinnamon or nutmeg to your regular tea or coffee. Try a dash of vanilla extract instead of sweetener as a zero-calorie addition to tea.

6. "Dietetic" on a label does not mean "diabetic." These foods are reduced in calories, but still may not be freely used. There are many variations. The sodium content may be low, but the sugar content high, or the sugar content low while the fat content is high. Read the labels.

7. If you buy canned fruit, purchase only the unsweetened kind packed in its own juice. Fresh fruit is best; it has not gone through processing which can cause the loss of vitamins and minerals.

8. Ideally, you should not buy packaged cookies, desserts, or mixes. They compromise nutrition for empty calories. Homemade breads, nuts, and fruits can satisfy your sweet tooth and wean you away from artificial sweeteners and processed products. But if you do buy processed or packaged items, always read the labels. In addition to brown sugar, sugar, corn syrup, corn sweeteners, honey, and molasses, dextrose, lactose, glucose, sorbitol, and mannitol are all forms of sugar. These packaged foods and mixes can also contain unnecessary amounts of fats and sodium.

9. Buy sugar-free tomato sauce or make your own. In these recipes, you will find that a small amount goes a long way. If used indiscriminately, the calories can add up fast. One-quarter cup of tomato sauce equals 70 to 80 calories.

10. Beware of artificial sweeteners. Instead, try to reduce your craving for sugar. Not one study has shown that artificial sweeteners help diabetics control their blood sugar or that they help dieters lose weight. In fact, some studies have shown that saccharin, for example, may actually stimulate the appetite and interfere with blood-sugar regulation. There is a cancer warning on products containing saccharin. In this world full of cancer-causing substances, don't increase your chances.

11. If you buy fruit juice, pay attention to the name of the drink. The name "fruit juice" must by law contain 100 percent real fruit juice; a "juice drink" can have anywhere from 35 to 69 percent real juice; a "fruit drink" may contain only 10 to 34 percent juice; and a "fruit-flavored drink" which has less than 10 percent juice may often have no juice at all. Water, sugar, flavorings, and coloring make up the rest of the drink.

12. Co-ops and bulk food buying clubs are a good place for the vegetarian to shop. They provide a wide variety of foods at low prices. Most co-ops and natural food stores keep their produce in bins or crocks. You can scoop out as much as you need. Buy only enough to last a week or two. Unpreserved, unrefined grains, wheat germ, other cereals, nuts, and seeds contain nutritious oils and should be refrigerated in a closed container to protect them from rancidity and mold.

13. Remember: Eat on time.

    Eat the proper amount for your diet
    Eat simple, nutritious foods.

Exercise

Exercise is important for a person with diabetes, because exercise is similar to taking a shot of insulin. Muscles that are being exercised need glucose from the blood which can reduce, or in some cases eliminate, the need for insulin or oral drugs, at least in the case of NIDDM.

People with IDDM, type-1 diabetes, also need exercise. Exercise can reduce the requirement for insulin intake. On the day of planned exercise, bring along snacks to prevent hypoglycemia. It is important to pay attention to your body and to always gradually increase the amount of exercise, taking into consideration how much exercise you can handle for the amount of insulin taken. Be careful.

To plan for extra caloric consumption when exercising,

Less than one hour of exercise: add 1 bread exchange.

One hour of exercise: add 1 bread and one protein exchange

Besides the immediate effect of clearing the blood of glucose, exercise has the long-term effect of increasing the body's sensitivity to insulin, especially in people with adult diabetes. Exercise keeps the blood thinner, which helps prevent blood clots.

The least painful method and the best way to begin exercising is by walking. Take the dog, your husband, wife, friend, or just go by yourself, and feel the freedom and relaxation of being able to go wherever your feet take you. While walking, you can plan your day, unwind from the day, think out a problem, or just take a break from your daily schedule. You will most likely be more energized and clear-headed than if you had taken a nap. This is a good way to start and may spur you onto serious hiking, or to take up skating, skiing, or some other physical activity. Don't give up. Find something you enjoy, and remember, using your body is the best way to keep it healthy.

Be sure to consult with your doctor before undertaking an exercise program.

Converting to a Vegetarian Diet

In the first edition of this book, I tried to replace meat exchanges with the protein in grains, nuts, beans, and seeds. Recent studies have shown that the kinds of calories consumed are as important as the amount of calories consumed.

The traditional exchange system breakdown used to consists of a diet that was 40% carbohydrate calories, 18% protein calories, and 41% fat calories. Now the American Diabetic Association has changed its recommendation to a lower fat content. Along with the emphasis on more fiber, a diet that is 60% complex carbohydrates, 30% fat, and 20% protein is now recommended.

The recipes in this book have been revised to reflect the lower fat diet that is now encouraged for people with diabetes. The exchanges will still be included, but I would encourage you to become aware of the composition of the foods you eat. If you do this, you will find it easier to eat a healthy diet and to control your diabetes.

Figuring Out Food Composition

The first step is to understand the following:

Carbohydrates have 4 calories per gram.

Protein has 4 calories per gram.

Fats have 9 calories per gram.

Alcohol has 7 calories per gram.

To figure out the percentage of protein, fat, or carbohydrates in a food the formula is:

The number of grams of carbohydrates, protein, or fat times the calories per gram, divided by the total number of calories in the recipe. The answer is the percentage of carbohydrates, protein, or fat in the recipe.

Recipe Example:

Cinnamon Raisin Muffins

Ingredients	Calories	Carbohydrates	Protein	Fat
2 cups whole wheat flour	800	160 gm.	30 gm.	4 gm.
1 ½ oz. raisins	107	26 gm.	1 gm.	--
½ cup walnuts	459	9 gm.	16 gm.	38 gm.
¼ cup oil	480	--	--	52 gm.
1 Tbsp. honey	65	16 gm.	--	--
Totals	**1911**	**211 gm.**	**47 gm.**	**94 gm.**

Carbohydrates are 211 grams x 4 calories per gram = 844
    divided by (the total number of calories) 1911 = 44% of calories
    from carbohydrates.

Menu Planning

This 5-day menu is based on a low-fat 1400-1600 calories diet. Each person with diabetes will be given a suggested amount of calories for the day's meals. Your diet may contain fewer calories or some may be much higher than the menu here, so be sure to get the correct calorie/insulin or oral medication ratio from your doctor.

	Breakfast 350-400 cal.	**Lunch** 450-500 cal.	**Dinner** 500-550 cal.	**Snack** 100-150 cal.
day one	hot oatmeal 1 orange	Tofu-Pita Pizza Free Green Salad Apple-Oat Cookies (2)	Three Bean Delight Quinoa Pilaf silced tomatoes Basic Whole Wheat Bread (one slice) soy margarine (1 tsp.)	popcorn (3 cups)
day two	Tofu French Toast (3) grapefruit (½)	Pat's Hummas Basic Whole Wheat Bread (2 slices) Non-fat Carrot Salad	Walnut-Lentil Loaf steamed kale Free Green Salad One Calorie Herb Dressing (1 tsp.) Eggless Rye Biscuit (1)	Tropical Fruit Salad

	Breakfast 350-400 cal.	**Lunch** 450-500 cal.	**Dinner** 500-550 cal.	**Snack** 100-150 cal.
day three	Whole Wheat Blueberry Hotcakes (3) cantalope (½)	Tofu "Egg Salad Style" (2 servings) Herbal Wheat Rolls (2) Quick-Rice Pudding apple (1 small)	Soybean-Mushroom Pilaf Green Peas Free Green Salad Lemon-Tomato Dressing Herb Roll (1) soy margarine (1 tsp.)	Strawberry Muffin (1) soymilk (½ cup)
day four	Banana-nog Basic Whole Wheat Bread (1 slice, toasted) soy margarine (1 tsp.)	Pea Soup Egg-less Rye Biscuits (2) Northern Fruit Salad	Vegetables w/ Stir-Fry Tofu brown rice (1 cup) Sesame Cornmeal Biscuit (1) soy margarine (1 tsp.)	Apple-Oat Drop Cookies (2)
day five	Scrambled Tofu English Muffin (1) soy margarine (1 tsp.) tomato or orange juice (4 Oz.)	The "Energizer"	Oven Eggplant whole wheat pasta (1 cup cooked) Free Green Salad Tahini Dressing	banana (1) Raisin Bran Biscuit

Cooking Chart for Grains and Beans

1 Cup Dry	Cups of Water	Cooking Time (Hours)	Yield (cups)
Barley	3	1	3.5
Black Beans	4	1.5	2
Black-Eyed Peas	3	1	2
Brown Rice	2	1	3
Buckwheat	2	15 min.	2.5
Bulgur	2	15 min.	2.5
Garbanzo Beans	4	2	2
Great Northern Beans	3	2	2
Kidney Beans	3	1.5	2
Lentils & Split Peas	3	1	2.25
Lima Beans	2	1.5	1.25
Millet	3	45 min.	3.5
Navy Beans	3	2.5	2
Oatmeal	2	5 min.	1.5
Pinto Beans	3	2.5	2
Soy Beans	3	pressure cook only 1 hour	2
Soy Grits	4	15 min.	2

Always cook your beans until they are soft.

Breakfast

Buckwheat Pancakes

Makes 8 pancakes

Mix together in a medium bowl:

1 ½ cups buckwheat flour
1 ½ tsps. baking powder

Beat in:

2 ¼ cups low-fat soymilk
1 Tbsp. oil

Heat lightly oiled frying pan on medium-high. When pan is hot, drop on by table-spoons. Flip once when bubbles appear, and cook until golden brown on bottom.

Per pancake: Calories: 112, 1 bread, ½ milk,
 Protein: 5 gm., Fat: 2 gm., Carbohydrates: 19 gm., Percentage of calories from fat: 20%

Cornmeal-Soy Pancakes

Makes 12 pancakes

Mix together in a medium bowl:
> **¾ cup whole wheat pastry flour**
> **¼ cup soy flour**
> **½ cup cornmeal**
> **2 tsps. baking powder**

Beat in:
> **2 cups low-fat soymilk**
> **1 Tbsp. oil**

Heat lightly oiled frying pan on medium-high. When pan is hot, drop on by table-spoons. Flip once when bubbles appear, and cook until golden brown on bottom.

Per pancake: Calories: 89, 1 bread,
> *Protein: 3 gm., Fat: 3 gm., Carbohydrates: 12 gm., Percentage of calories from fat: 33%*

The Energizer

One serving

Toss together:
> **1 Tbsp. cashews**
> **1 Tbsp. sunflower seeds**
> **2 Tbsps. wheat germ**
> **½ cup oatmeal**
> **2 tsps. chopped dates**

Put in a dessert bowl:
> **½ cup soy yogurt**

Top with:
> **the nut mixture**
> **½ banana, sliced**

Per serving: Calories: 516, 2 breads, 1 milk, 3 fats, 2 fruit
> *Protein: 21 gm., Fat: 17 gm., Carbohydrates: 64 gm., Percentage of calories from fat: 28%*

Oatmeal Pancakes

Makes 8 pancakes

These pancakes are great for lunch sandwiches too.
Oatmeal ones are especially good with peanut butter.

Mix together in a medium bowl:
- **1½ cups oatmeal**
- **½ cup whole wheat flour**
- **2 tsps. baking powder**
- **1 tsp. cinnamon**

Beat in:
- **1¼ cups low-fat soymilk**
- **1 Tbsp. oil**
- **¼ cup raisins**

Heat lightly oiled frying pan on medium-high. When pan is hot, drop on by table-spoons. Flip once when bubbles appear, and cook until golden brown on bottom.

Per pancake: Calories: 148, 1 bread, ½ fruit, ½ milk,
Protein: 5 gm., Fat: 2 gm., Carbohydrates: 25 gm., Percentage of calories from fat: 18%

Raisin-Rice Cakes

Makes 10 pancakes

A delicious pancake recipe without oil.

Mix together in a medium bowl:
>   **1½ cups whole wheat pastry flour**
>   **1 cup cooked rice**
>   **1½ tsps. baking powder**
>   **1 tsp. cinnamon**

Beat in:
>   **1¾ cups low-fat soymilk**

Stir in:
>   **¼ cup raisins**

Heat lightly oiled frying pan on medium-high. When pan is hot, drop on by table-spoons. Flip once when bubbles appear, and cook until golden brown on bottom.

Per pancake: Calories: 107, 1 bread, ½ milk,
  Protein: 3 gm., Fat: 0 gm., Carbohydrates: 22 gm., Percentage of calories from fat: 6%

Scrambled Tofu

One serving

Sauté together:
>   **½ tsp. oil**
>   **1 slice onion**
>   **a little water if needed**

Add and scramble until hot:
>   **4 oz. reduced-fat tofu, crumbled**
>   **1 tsp. herb mix**
>   **¼ tsp. curry**

Per serving: Calories: 142, 1½ meat, ½ fat
  Protein: 13 gm., Fat: 7 gm., Carbohydrates: 7 gm., Percentage of calories from fat: 46%

Tofu French Toast

Makes 6 pieces of toast

Mix in blender until smooth:
>**8 oz. low-fat tofu**
>**½ cup water**
>**1 tsp. honey**
>**½ tsp. cinnamon**
>**1 banana**

Pour blended mixture into a shallow dish. Dip into mixture:
>**6 slices whole wheat bread**

Cook on a non-stick pan.

Each slice: Calories: 107, 1 bread, ½ fruit,
Protein: 4 gm., Fat: 0 gm., Carbohydrates: 17 gm., Percentage of calories from fat: 12%

Whole Wheat Blueberry Pancakes

Makes 12 pancakes

Mix together in a medium bowl:
>**2 cups whole wheat flour**
>**2 tsps. baking powder**

Beat in:
>**2¼ cups low-fat soymilk**
>**1 Tbsp. oil**

Stir in:
>**1 cup blueberries**

Heat lightly oiled frying pan on medium-high. When pan is hot, drop on by table-spoons. Flip once when bubbles appear, and cook until golden brown on bottom.

Per pancake: Calories: 101, 1 bread, ½ milk, ½ fat
Protein: 3 gm., Fat: 2 gm., Carbohydrates: 18 gm., Percentage of calories from fat: 17%

Breakfast in the Blender

These drinks are a nutritious and satisfying way to start the day. If you add a couple of bread exchanges, breakfast can seem like a feast!

Banana - Nogg

One serving

Blend in a blender until smooth and creamy:

1 cup low-fat soymilk
1 Tbsp. low-fat soymilk powder
1 tsp. vanilla
1 banana
pinch of cinnamon or nutmeg

Per serving: Calories: 259, 1½ milk, 2 fruit
Protein: 6 gm., Fat: 3 gm., Carbohydrates: 47 gm., Percentage of calories from fat: 8%

Creamy Peanut and Pineapple Shake

One serving

This one is good with any juice or without the juice. Without the juice, you will be able to have a piece of fruit if your diet plan allows it at that meal.

Blend in a blender until smooth and creamy:

1 cup low-fat soymilk
¼ cup low-fat soymilk powder
1 Tbsp. peanut butter
½ tsp. vanilla
⅛ cup pincapple juice

Per serving: Calories: 380, 2 milk, 1 meat, 1 fruit, 2 fat
Protein: 12 gm., Fat: 9 gm., Carbohydrates: 57 gm., Percentage of calories from fat: 21%

Cereals

Instead of corn flakes or cream of wheat, try adding other grains to your breakfast menu. Bulgur, millet, oats, buckwheat, brown rice, rye or wheat flakes, and barley can all be prepared for breakfast. Here are a few favorite combinations:

✢

Brown Rice
One serving

Bring to a boil in a small saucepan:
> **⅔ cup water**
> **⅓ cup brown rice**

Simmer covered for 30 minutes. Remove from heat.

Add:
> **2 chopped figs**
> **¼ tsp. nutmeg**

Serve in a bowl with:
> **¼ cup low-fat soymilk or soy yogurt**

Per serving: Calories: 270, 2 breads, 1 fruit, 1 milk
Protein: 5 gm., Fat: 1 gm., Carbohydrates: 59 gm., Percentage of calories from fat: 5%

Baked Oatmeal

Two servings

Preheat oven to 350°F.

Oil a small casserole dish with:
>   **1 tsp. oil**

Mix together in the caserole in the order listed:
>   **1½ cups oatmeal**
>   **2 Tbsps. low-fat soymilk powder**
>   **1 banana, mashed**
>   **1½ cups hot water**

Bake for 20 minutes.

Per serving: Calories: 346, 1 milk, 2½ breads, 2 fats, 1 fruit
*   Protein: 9 gm., Fat: 10 gm., Carbohydrates: 54 gm., Percentage of calories from fat: 27%*

Variation

Replace banana with:
>   **2 Tbsps. raisins**
>   **¼ cup coconut**

Sprinkle with:
>   **cinnamon**

Bake for 20 minutes.

Per serving: Calories: 507, 1 milk, 2½ breads, 3 fats, 2 fruit
*   Protein: 12 gm., Fat: 23 gm., Carbohydrates: 61 gm., Percentage of calories from fat: 40%*

Bulgur Wheat

One serving

Bring to a boil in a small saucepan:
⅔ cup water
⅓ cup bulgur wheat

Simmer, covered, until liquid is absorbed.

Blend to a fine powder in a blender:
2 Tbsps. cashews

Add and blend again:
½ tsp. vanilla
¼ cup low-fat soymilk or soy yogurt

Pour over bulgur and cook 5 more minutes. Add:
1 banana, sliced

Per serving: Calories: 466, 2½ breads, 1 fruit, 2 fats, 1 milk
Protein: 13 gm., Fat: 9 gm., Carbohydrates: 82 gm., Percentage of calories from fat: 10%

Granola

Makes 7 cups

Oatmeal is the one grain which does not have to be cooked to be digested.
By not cooking it, no vitamins are lost.

Mix together and store in an airtight container in the refrigerator:
3 cups rolled oats
½ cup bran
½ cup wheat germ
½ cup raisins, chopped
½ cup dates, chopped
1 cup almonds, chopped
2 Tbsps. sesame seed

Per ½ cup: Calories: 198, 1 bread, 1 fruit, 2 fats
Protein: 6 gm., Fat: 7 gm., Carbohydrates: 26 gm., Percentage of calories from fat: 34%

Hot Oatmeal

One serving

Mix in a small pan:
1 cup hot water
⅔ cup oatmeal

Cook gently for 5 to 6 minutes.

Add:
1 Tbsp. raisins
½ tsp. cinnamon
1 Tbsp. sunflower seeds

Serve with:
¼ cup low-fat soymilk or soy yogurt

Per serving: Calories: 324, 2 breads, 1 fruit, 1 fat, 1 milk
Protein: 13 gm., Fat: 8 gm., Carbohydrates: 57 gm., Percentage of calories from fat: 24%

Breads

Banana – Raisin Bran Biscuits

Makes 12 biscuits

Preheat oven to 350°F.

Mix together in a medium mixing bowl:
> **1 ½ cups whole wheat pastry flour**
> **½ cup bran**
> **2 tsps. baking powder**

Stir in:
> **½ cup low-fat soymilk**
> **1 tsp. vanilla**
> **1 banana, mashed**

Add:
> **½ cup raisins**
> **½ cup chopped walnuts**

Drop onto ungreased cookie sheet, making 12 biscuits.

Bake for 15 minutes.

Per biscuit: Calories: 119, 1 bread, 1 fruit
  Protein: 3 gm., Fat: 3 gm., Carbohydrates: 19 gm., Percentage of calories: from fat: 23%

Basic Whole Wheat Bread

Makes 2 loaves

A little bit of honey in a yeast bread makes the bread rise better. One tablespoon in a loaf of bread does not contribute significant calories. The bread can be made without it, but if you are new to working with whole wheat, you may find that you need help in getting it to rise the first few times. A little honey to help the yeast may be all you will need.

Stir together in a large bowl until the yeast is dissolved:
> **1 Tbsp. honey**
> **1 Tbsp. yeast**
> **2½ cups warm water**

Beat in:
> **3 cups whole wheat flour**

Mix in gradually:
> **3 additional cups whole wheat flour**

On a lightly floured surface, knead the dough until it is soft and springy. Form into 2 loaves and place in two lightly oiled 9" x 5" bread pans. Cover the pans with a clean towel. Let the bread rise until almost double in size. Bake at 350°F for 45 minutes.

15 slices per loaf, each slice: Calories: 83, 1 bread
    Protein: 3 gm., Fat: 0 gm., Carbohydrates: 17 gm., Percentage of calories: from fat: 4%

The Best English Muffins

Makes twelve 4" muffins

This is our favorite bread. We like them best split and toasted.

Combine and set aside:
> **2 Tbsps. yeast**
> **½ cup flour**

Heat in a small saucepan until warm:
> **1¾ cups low-fat soymilk**
> **1 Tbsp. honey (optional)**
> **2 Tbsps. oil**

Stir the yeast and flour into the milk mixture, and mix until dissolved. Pour this into a large bowl.

Beat in:
> **4 cups whole wheat or unbleached flour**

Knead ten minutes on a lightly floured surface. Roll out the dough and cut into twelve 4-inch rounds. Place the rounds on a floured baking sheet.

Let rise one hour. Bake at 350°F for about 25 minutes.

Per muffin: Calories: 187, 2 breads, 1 fat
Protein: 7 gm., Fat: 2 gm., Carbohydrates: 33 gm., Percentage of calories: from fat: 10%

Blueberry Oat Muffins

Makes 12 muffins

Preheat oven to 350°F.

Mix together in a medium mixing bowl:
>   **1 cup whole wheat flour**
>   **1 cup rolled oats**
>   **½ tsp. cinnamon**
>   **1 Tbsp. baking powder**

Stir in carefully and avoid over mixing:
>   **1 cup low-fat soymilk**
>   **1 Tbsp. honey**
>   **2 Tbsps. oil**

Fold in:
>   **1 cup blueberries**

Spoon into lightly oiled muffin cups. Bake 15-20 minutes.

Per muffin: Calories: 101, 1 bread, ½ fat,
>   *Protein: 3 gm., Fat: 3 gm., Carbohydrate: 15 gm., Percentage of calories: from fat: 27%*

Bran and Wheat Germ Muffins

Makes 12 muffins

The addition of a banana gives plenty of natural sweetness to these muffins without a lot of calories.

Preheat oven to 375°F.

Mix together in a medium mixing bowl:

1 cup whole wheat pastry flour
½ cup bran
½ cup wheat germ
1½ tsps. cinnamon
2 tsps. baking powder

Stir in and avoid over mixing:

¼ cup low-fat soymilk powder
¼ cup water
2 Tbsps. oil
1 banana, mashed

Fold in:

⅓ cup chopped walnuts

Spoon into lightly oiled muffin cups. Bake for 15-20 minutes.

Per muffin: Calories: 122, 1 bread, 1 fat
Protein: 4 gm., Fat: 7 gm., Carbohydrates: 15 gm., Percentage of calories: from fat: 35%

Cinnamon Raisin Muffins

Makes 12 muffins

Preheat oven to 400°F

Mix together:

       2 cups whole wheat pastry flour
       2 tsps. baking powder
       1 tsp. cinnamon

Stir in:

       1½ oz. raisins (¼ cup)
       ½ cup walnuts
       1¾ cups water
       ¼ cup oil
       1 Tbsp. honey

Stir liquids into dry ingredients, being careful not to over mix. Spoon into oiled muffin tins. Bake for 15 minutes.

Per muffin: Calories: 159, 1 bread, 2 fats
    Protein: 4 gm., Fat: 8 gm., Carbohydrates: 17 gm., Percentage of calories: from fat: 44%

Cornmeal Rice Buns

Makes 9 buns

Preheat oven to 375°F.

Combine in a medium bowl, stirring until smooth:
- **1 cup boiling water**
- **1¼ cups cornmeal**
- **2 Tbsps. soy flour**

Mix in:
- **1 cup cooked rice**
- **2 Tbsps. oil**

Form 9 patties. Bake on floured baking sheet 25-30 minutes.

Per bun: Calories: 129, 1 bread, 1 fat
Protein: 3 gm., Fat: 3 gm., Carbohydrates: 21 gm., Percentage of calories: from fat: 21%

Egg – less Rye Biscuits

Makes 12 biscuits

Preheat oven 350°F.

Mix together in a medium mixing bowl:
- **2 cups light rye flour**
- **2 tsps. baking powder**

Stir in:
- **1 cup low-fat soymilk**
- **2 Tbsps. oil**

Spoon onto lightly oiled cookie sheet, making 12 biscuits. Bake for 10-15 minutes.

Per biscuit: Calories: 98, 1 bread, ½ fat
Protein: 3 gm., Fat: 2 gm., Carbohydrates: 15 gm., Percentage of calories: from fat: 18%

Half Whole Wheat Bread

Makes 2 loaves

Dissolve together:
4 tsps. dry yeast
1 cup lukewarm water
1 tsp. honey

Set aside for 10 minutes.

Combine and set aside:
4 cups whole wheat flour
3 cups white unbleached flour

Mix together in a large bowl:
¼ cup honey
⅓ cup oil
2 cups warm low-fat soymilk
the yeast mixture

Stir the flour mixture into the liquid ingredients in the large bowl to make a kneadable dough. Turn the dough onto a floured surface, and knead for 10 minutes, adding more white flour if dough is too wet. Divide dough in half and place each half in a lightly oiled 9" x 5" bread pan . Cover pans with a towel, and let the dough rise for 1½ hours. Bake at 350°F for 1 hour or until done.

One loaf about 16 large slices, each slice: Calories: 122, 1½ bread or 1 bread, ½ low-fat milk Protein: 3 gm., Fat: 2 gm., Carbohydrates: 21 gm., Percentage of calories: from fat: 15%

Herbed Wheat Rolls

Makes 10 rolls

These little buns are great for accompanying a salad or a vegetable soup.

Preheat oven to 350°F.

Heat in a small saucepan until warm:

1 cup low-fat soymilk

Add:

1 Tbsp. yeast
2 tsps. canola oil

Beat in:

1½ cups whole wheat flour
½ tsp. dill
½ tsp. oregano
½ tsp. thyme

Drop by tablespoons onto floured baking sheet, making 10 rolls. Bake about 15 minutes.

Per roll: Calories: 80, 1 bread
　　Protein: 3 gm., Fat: 2 gm., Carbohydrates: 14 gm., Percentage of calories: from fat: 23%

Nutritional Yeast Gravy or Sauce

Makes 2½ cups

Combine in a saucepan:
>   **⅓ cup nutritional yeast**
>   **⅓ cup flour**
>   **2 cups water**

Cook over low heat until bubbling. Remove from heat.

Add:
>   **1 Tbsp. soy margarine**
>   **1 tsp. prepared mustard**

For a darker sauce, mix the flour and yeast in a saucepan, and brown first.

Per 2 Tbsps.: Calories: 20, ¼ bread (If you use a half cup per serving add 1 fat)
*   Protein: 1 gm., Fat: 0 gm., Carbohydrates: 2 gm., Percentage of calories: from fat: 24%*

Orange Cranberry Muffins

Makes 12 muffins

Pictured on the cover.

Preheat oven to 350°F.

Mix together in a medium bowl:
> **¾ cup whole wheat flour**
> **¾ cup unbleached white flour**
> **½ cup oats, coarsely ground in a blender**
> **½ Tbsp. baking powder**
> **½ Tbsp. baking soda**
> **½ tsp. cinnamon**

Blend together:
> **¾ cup orange juice**
> **½ Tbsp. vanilla**
> **¼ cup unsweetened applesauce**
> **6 oz. low-fat tofu**

Add carefully to dry ingredients to avoid over mixing.

Fold in:
> **½ cup dehydrated cranberries**

Bake in a lightly oiled or non-stick muffin cups for 20-25 minutes.

Raisins can be substituted for the cranberries.

Per muffin: Calories: 81, 1 bread
Protein: 3 gm., Fat: 0 gm., Carbohydrate: 15 gm., Percentage of calories: from fat: 5%

Raisin Tofu Scones

Makes 10 scones

Preheat oven to 350°F.

Sift together:

1 cup whole wheat flour
1 cup unbleached white flour
2 tsps. baking powder

Add:

4 oz. low-fat tofu, mashed
1 cup low-fat soymilk
2 Tbsps. honey
1 tsp. vanilla
½ cup raisins

Mix well. Roll out on a floured surface. Cut into 10 triangles. Bake for 15 minutes.

Per scone: 128 Calories: 1 bread, 1 fruit
Protein: 3 gm., Fat: 0 gm., Carbohydrate: 26 gm., Percentage of calories: from fat: 4%

Sesame-Cornmeal Biscuits

Makes 12 biscuits

Preheat oven to 350°F.

Mix together thoroughly in a medium mixing bowl:
> **1 cup whole wheat pastry flour**
> **⅔ cup cornmeal**
> **⅓ cup wheat germ**
> **2 tsps. baking powder**
> **1 Tbsp. sesame seeds**

Add and beat well:
> **1 Tbsp. oil**
> **1 cup low-fat soymilk**

Drop onto floured cookie sheet by tablespoons, making 12 biscuits. Bake 20-25 minutes.

Per biscuit: Calories: 95, 1 bread, ½ fat
> *Protein: 3 gm., Fat: 2 gm., Carbohydrates: 15 gm., Percentage of calories: from fat: 19%*

Strawberry Muffins

Makes 12 muffins

Preheat oven to 350°F.

Mix together in a medium bowl:
> **1 cup whole wheat pastry flour**
> **1 cup oats, coarsely ground in a blender**
> **½ tsp. cinnamon**
> **2 tsps. baking powder**

Blend together:
> **1 Tbsp. honey**
> **¼ cup low-fat soymilk**
> **12 oz. low-fat tofu**
> **3 Tbsps. unsweetened applesauce**
> **1 tsp. vanilla**

Add carefully to dry ingredients to avoid over mixing.

Fold in:
> **½ cup strawberries, sliced**

Bake in a lightly oiled or non-stick muffin cups for 20 - 25 minutes.

Per muffin: Calories: 84, 1 bread,
Protein: 3 gm., Fat: 0 gm., Carbohydrate: 13 gm., Percentage of calories: from fat: 9%

Salads

✛

Basic Free Green Salad

Enjoy up to 2 cups free! Pictured on the cover.

2 cups shredded romaine lettuce
2 cups shredded iceberg lettuce
1 cup curly endive
1 cup shredded spinach or Swiss chard
12 sliced or whole radishes
1 cucumber, sliced
2 stalks celery, diced, with tops

Other ingredients to form your own combinations:

Boston or bibb lettuce
shredded red or green cabbage
kale or comfrey
chicory or sorrel
lamb's-quarters leaves
parsley or watercress
turnip, collard, mustard,
   dandelion, or beet greens
green or wax beans
onions, tomatoes, sprouts
sliced fresh mushrooms
sliced fresh red or green peppers
flowerets of broccoli or cauliflower
slices of zucchini or yellow squash
brussels sprouts, halved or quartered
scallions or chives

Garbanzo - Noodle Salad With Yogurt

Two servings

Mix together:

1 cup cooked garbanzos
2 cups cooked whole wheat noodles
2 Tbsps. onions, chopped
1 cup broccoli, chopped and steamed until just tender
1 cup carrots, chopped and steamed
1 Tbsp. sesame tahini
1 Tbsp. lemon juice
2 tsps. Herb Mix (page 138)

Top with:

½ cup plain soy yogurt

Per serving: Calories: 521, 2 meats, 2 breads, 2 vegetables, 1 fat
Protein: 21 gm., Fat: 8 gm., Carbohydrates: 81 gm., Percentage of calories from fat: 15%

Non-Fat Carrot Salad

Two servings

Mix together:
>**1 cup carrots, grated**
>**½ apple, grated**
>**¼ cup raisins**

Soaked in:
>**2 Tbsps. orange juice**
>**1 tsp. lemon juice**

Refrigerate for at least a half day.

Per serving: Calories: 105, 1 vegetable, 1½ fruit
>*Protein: 1 gm., Fat: 0 gm., Carbohydrates: 25 gm., Percentage of calories from fat: 1%*

Patty's Tabouli

Eight servings

Bring water to boil. Add bulgur. Remove from heat and set aside for ½ hour.
>**4 cups water**
>**2 cups bulgur wheat**

Put cooked bulgur into a salad bowl, and mix in rest of ingredients:
>**2 cups tomatoes, chopped**
>**2 Tbsps. olive oil**
>**2 cloves garlic, minced**
>**3 Tbsps. chives, chopped**
>**½ cup parsley, chopped**
>**1 Tbsp. lemon juice**
>**salt & pepper to taste**

Refrigerate overnight.

Per serving: Calories: 182, 1½ bread, 1 vegetable, ½ fat
>*Protein: 6 gm., Fat: 3 gm., Carbohydrates: 32 gm., Percentage of calories from fat: 17%*

Rice Salad

Six servings

Combine all ingredients and mix well:

4 cups brown rice, cooked
1 cup onion, finely chopped
1 cup celery, finely chopped
1 cup carrot, grated
1 cup alfalfa sprouts
2 cups cooked garbanzo beans
2 cups tomato, finely chopped
3 Tbsps. olive oil
1 Tbsp. cider vinegar
½ tsp. salt
1 Tbsp. mixed herbs, such as basil, parley, garlic powder, oregano, thyme etc. (see recipe page 138)

Per serving: Calories: 344, 2 meat, 1 bread, 2 fat, 1 vegetable
Protein: 9 gm., Fat: 8 gm., Carbohydrates: 58 gm., Percentage of calories from fat: 21%

Sprouts

These beans and seeds can be sprouted.

wheat or rye berries   mung beans
sunflower seeds   soybeans
sesame seeds   lentils
alfalfa seeds   watercress seeds
radish seeds   garbanzo beans

Rinse beans or seeds, put about 2 Tbsps. in a quart jar with water, and let soak overnight or at least 6 hours. Cover top with cheese cloth or sprouting jar cover (which can be found in many department stores). After the soaking time is up, drain the water through the covers or cloth. Rinse two or three times a day to keep sprouts moist. Drain completely after each rinse to prevent decay. They will begin to sprout in one or two days and will be fully sprouted in 4 or 5 days. Keep them in the refrigerator after they are fully sprouted, and use promptly.

Three-Bean Delight

Four servings

Toss together:

    1 cup cooked kidney beans
    1 cup cooked garbanzo beans
    1 cup cooked lima beans
    1 cup onion, chopped
    ½ cup green pepper, chopped
    4 tsps. olive oil

Serve hot or cold with a grain or bread. To serve cold for a salad, add a few drops of lemon juice or vinegar.

Per serving: Calories: 236, 2½ meats, 1 fat
    Protein: 10 gm., Fat: 6 gm., Carbohydrates: 36 gm., Percentage of calories from fat: 20%

Tofu Potato Salad

One serving

This tofu salad makes a great hot weather dish.

Steam and dice:
> **1 large potato (1 cup)**

Mix together in a medium bowl with the diced potato:
> **6 oz. low- fat tofu, diced**
> **½ cup diced tomato**
> **2 Tbsps. onion, chopped**
> **2 Tbsps. pepper, chopped**
> **½ cup alfalfa sprouts**
> **½ tsp. oregano**
> **¼ tsp. rosemary**
> **1 tsp. tarragon**
> **¼ tsp. ground bay leaves**
> **¼ tsp. basil**
> **1 Tbsp. sunflower seeds**
> **1 oz. unsalted peanuts**
> **1 tsp. low-fat soy mayonnaise**

Serve on a bed of lettuce.

Per serving: Calories: 469, 3 meats, 2 breads, 2 fats, 1 vegetable
Protein: 15 gm., Fat: 18 gm., Carbohydrates: 42 gm., Percentage of calories from fat: 36%

Tofu Salad 1

Two servings

Mix together:

>   **10.5 oz. low-fat tofu, diced**
>   **½ cup tomato, chopped**
>   **¼ cup peppers and onions, chopped**

Place on a bed of lettuce, and garnish with cucumber slices and alfalfa sprouts. Use **Lemon-Tomato Juice Dressing** (page 79) or **One-Calorie Herb Dressing** (page 79).

Per serving: Calories: 66, ½ meat, 1 vegetable
  Protein: 3 gm., Fat: 0 gm., Carbohydrates: 3 gm., Percentage of calories from fat: 7%

Tofu Salad 2

One serving

Mix together:

>   **6 oz. tofu, diced**
>   **1 Tbsp. tahini**

Stir in:

>   **½ cup tomato, chopped**
>   **¼ cup peppers and onions, chopped**
>   **¼ cup carrots, finely diced**
>   **¼ cup sprouts**

Place on a bed of lettuce.

Per serving: Calories: 215, 1 meat, 2 fats, 2 vegetables
  Protein: 8 gm., Fat: 8 gm., Carbohydrates: 11 gm., Percentage of calories from fat: 34%

Vegetarian "Chef's Salad"

One serving

Any of the dressings are good with this salad, but our favorite is the tahini.

Mix in a large individual salad bowl:
> **2 cups Basic Free Green Salad (page 70)**

Add:
> **¼ cup low-fat tofu diced**
> **¼ cup cold garbanzo beans**
> **2 Tbsps. peanuts**

Top with:
> **1 slice toasted whole wheat bread, cut into crouton-sized cubes**

Per serving: Calories: 300, 3 meat, 1 fat, 1 bread
Protein: 16 gm., Fat: 11 gm., Carbohydrates: 31 gm., Percentage of calories from fat: 33%

Salad Dressings

✤

Herbed Olive Oil Dressing

Makes 1 cup

Mix together thoroughly:

⅓ cup olive oil
3 Tbsps. wine vinegar
2 Tbsps. parsley, chopped
¼ tsp. kelp powder
¼ tsp. pepper
enough water to make 1 cup

Per Tbsp.: Calories 38, 1 fat
Protein: 0 gm., Fat: 4 gm., Carbohydrates: 0 gm., Percentage of calories from fat: 94%

Herbed Yogurt Dressing

Makes 1 cup

Mix together thoroughly:

1 cup soy yogurt
4 Tbsps. chives
1 tsp. tarragon
1 tsp. dill
½ tsp. bay
½ tsp. basil
½ tsp. marjoram
1 Tbsp. lemon juice

1 Tbsp.: Free   Per Tbsp.: Calories: 10
Protein: 1 gm., Fat: 0 gm., Carbohydrates: 1 gm., Percentage of calories from fat: 26%

Lemon-Tomato Juice Dressing

Makes 1⅓ cups

Mix together thoroughly:
- **1 cup tomato juice**
- **2 Tbsps. lemon juice**
- **1 tsp. basil**
- **1 tsp. bay**
- **2 Tbsps. onion, chopped**
- **1 Tbsp. parsley, chopped**

1-3 Tbsp.: Free   Per Tbsp.: Calories: 3
Protein: 0 gm., Fat: 0 gm., Carbohydrates: 1 gm., Percentage of calories from fat: 0%

One-Calorie Herb Dressing

Makes 1 cup

Mix together thoroughly:
- **½ cup cider or wine vinegar**
- **½ cup water**
- **½ tsp. dry mustard**
- **½ tsp. pepper**
- **1 tsp. celery seed**
- **1 tsp. dill seed**

Free   Per Tbsp.: Calories: 1
Protein: 0 gm., Fat: 0 gm., Carbohydrates: 1 gm., Percentage of calories from fat: 0%

"Russian" Yogurt Dressing

Makes 1½ cups

Mix together thoroughly:
> **2 Tbsps. sugar-free ketchup**
> **1 cup soy yogurt**
> **¼ cup water**
> **1 clove garlic, minced**
> **2 Tbsps. dill pickle, chopped**
> **2 Tbsps. chives, chopped**
> **½ tsp. mustard powder**
> **½ tsp. tamari**

1 Tbsp.: Free   Per Tbsp.: Calories: 8
Protein: 1 gm., Fat: 0 gm., Carbohydrates: 1 gm., Percentage of calories from fat: 24%

Tahini Dressing

Makes 2 cups

Mix together thoroughly:
> **1 cup sesame tahini**
> **3 Tbsps. lemon juice**
> **⅔ cup water**
> **1 Tbsp. onion, minced**
> **1 clove garlic, minced**

Per Tbsp.: Calories: 55, 1 fat
Protein: 1 gm., Fat: 5 gm., Carbohydrates: 2 gm., Percentage of calories from fat: 69%

3

6 oz. tofu, diced
2 tsps. tahini
¼ cup alfalfa sprouts

Per sandwich: Calories: 136, 1½ meat, ½ fat
Protein: 5 gm., Fat: 6 gm., Carbohydrates: 4 gm., Percentage of calories from fat: 36%

4

2 oz. sliced tempeh, steamed 10 minutes
1 oz. soy cheese slice
slice of tomato

Per sandwich: Calories: 200, 2 meat, 1 fat
Protein: 12 gm., Fat: 11 gm., Carbohydrates: 12 gm., Percentage of calories from fat: 48%

Sandwiches

Four Great Bean Sandwiches

One serving each

These also make good sandwiches for traveling. The tempeh-tomato-soy cheese sandwich is good when heated in the oven.

1

¼ cup cooked pinto beans, mashed
2 tsps. tomato sauce
1 tsp. onion, chopped
2 Tbsps. soy cheddar cheese, grated
shredded lettuce

Per sandwich: Calories: 123, 1½ meat, ½ fat
Protein: 5 gm., Fat: 5 gm., Carbohydrates: 14 gm., Percentage of calories from fat: 35%

2

¼ cup cooked garbanzo beans, mashed
2 tsps. tahini
1 tsp. onion, chopped
pinch garlic powder
1 tsp. lemon juice

Per sandwich: Calories: 133, 1½ meat, ½ fat
Protein: 5 gm., Fat: 6 gm., Carbohydrates: 15 gm., Percentage of calories from fat: 38%

Crunchy Peanut Garbanzo Pitas

One serving

Mix together:

       ½ cup cooked garbanzo beans
       ½ cup celery, diced
       ¼ cup alfalfa sprouts
       2 Tbsps. peanuts
       2 tsps. tahini
       1 tsp. tamari

Slice open:

       1 (2 oz.) pita bread

Fill pita bread with crunchy peanut mix. Serve hot or cold.

Per sandwich: Calories: 465, 3 meat, 2 bread, 2 fat
    Protein: 19 gm., Fat: 16 gm., Carbohydrates: 58 gm., Percentage of calories from fat: 31%

Pat's Hummus

Four servings

Puree in blender until smooth:

2 cups garbanzo beans, cooked
2 Tbsps. tahini
1 Tbsp. lemon juice
1 Tbsp. water
1 Tbsp. olive oil
¼ cup onion, chopped
1 Tbsp. parsley, chopped

Makes filling for 4 sandwiches.

Per serving (without bread): Calories: 216, 1½ meat, 2 fats
Protein: 8 gm., Fat: 8 gm., Carbohydrates: 26 gm., Percentage of calories from fat: 35%

Ratatouille Pitas

One serving

Preheat oven to 325°F.

Simmer in a medium saucepan until tender:

1 Tbsp. onion, chopped
½ cup tomato, diced
½ cup zucchini or eggplant, diced
2 Tbsps. water

Remove from heat.

Mix in:

¼ cup soy cheddar cheese, grated
1 Tbsp. nutritional yeast

Slice open:

1 (2 oz.) pita bread

Fill the pita bread with ratatouille mix. Wrap in foil and heat in oven until thoroughly warm - about 5 minutes.

Spread on top:

¼ cup alfalfa sprouts

Per sandwich: Calories: 315, 1½ meat, 2 breads, 2 vegetables
Protein: 14 gm., Fat: 10 gm., Carbohydrates: 39 gm., Percentage of calories from fat: 31%

Tofu Pita Pizzas

One serving

Preheat oven to 325°F.

Separate into two halves and place on a baking sheet:
> **1 (2 oz.) pita bread**

Mix together:
> **6 oz. low-fat tofu, diced**
> **½ cup mushrooms, chopped**
> **4 thin slices onion**
> **4 thin slices green pepper**
> **2 Tbsps. tomato sauce**

Top with:
> **2 Tbsps. soy Parmesan**

Bake for 10 - 15 minutes.

Per two halves: Calories: 333, 2 meat, 2 breads, 1 vegetable
Protein: 20 gm., Fat: 2 gm., Carbohydrates: 45 gm., Percentage of calories from fat: 6%

Soups

✛

Creamy Garbanzo Soup

Four servings

Cook until the beans are soft (about 2 hours):

1 ½ cups garbanzo beans
2 cups onion, chopped
½ cup celery, chopped
½ cup carrots, diced
6 cups water

Puree in a blender, then return to the pot.

Stir in:

2 cups low-fat soymilk
¼ cup low-fat soymilk powder

Steam and add to the soup:

1 ½ cups carrots, diced

Season to taste with:

pepper, parsley, and kelp

Per serving: Calories: 336, 3½ meats, ½ bread, ½ milk
Protein: 13 gm., Fat: 3 gm., Carbohydrates: 60 gm., Percentage of calories from fat: 9%

Easy Lentil Stew

Six servings

Cook for about 1 hour:

1 cup lentils, uncooked
1 cup brown rice, uncooked
thyme, oregano, pepper to taste
6 cups water

Add more water if needed.

Add and cook another 15 minutes:

2 cups carrots, diced
1 cup onion, chopped
2 stalks celery with tops, diced
1 medium tomato, chopped
1 cup spinach, shredded (optional)

Per serving: Calories: 249, 2 meats, 1 bread, 2 vegetables
Protein: 11 gm., Fat: 0 gm., Carbohydrates: 49 gm., Percentage of calories from fat: 3%

Garbanzo-Vegetable Soup

One serving

Pictured on the cover.

Have ready:

½ cup cooked garbanzo beans

Bring to a boil in a 2 quart saucepan, cover, and simmer for 10 minutes:

½ cup fresh or frozen corn
½ cup fresh or frozen green beans
½ cup carrots, diced
½ cup celery, diced
1 cup shredded spinach or cabbage
¼ cup onions, chopped
2 cups water
½ tsp. each: parsley, oregano, basil, bay leaves to taste

Add:

1 tsp. tomato sauce
the cooked garbanzo beans
¼ cup uncooked whole wheat or enriched noodles

Simmer 5 more minutes, until noodles are cooked.

Per serving: Calories: 406, 3 meats, 2 breads, 2 vegetables
  Protein: 14 gm., Fat: 2 gm., Carbohydrates: 81 gm., Percentage of calories from fat: 4%

Kale Potato Soup

Six servings

Bring to a boil and cook until potatoes are soft:

5 cups water
1 large onion, chopped
2 cloves garlic, minced
3 medium potatoes, chopped
salt & pepper to taste

Add:

4 cups steamed kale, chopped

Remove half the soup and blend in the blender. Return blended mixture to the pot, and stir. Serve hot.

Per serving: Calories: 90, 1 vegetable, 1 bread
Protein: 2 gm., Fat: 0 gm., Carbohydrates: 20 gm., Percentage of calories from fat: 2%

Pea Soup

Four 1½ cup servings

Cook covered for 1 hour:

1 cup dried split peas
¼ cup barley, uncooked
6 cups of water

Add, cover, and cook another 30 minutes:

1 cup potato, diced
1 cup onions, chopped
1 cup cabbage, shredded
1 stalk celery, diced
1 cup carrots, diced
bay, basil, tarragon, pepper to taste

Per serving: Calories: 208, 2 meats, ½ breads, 2 vegetables
Protein: 9 gm., Fat: 0 gm., Carbohydrates: 42 gm., Percentage of calories from fat: 2%

Tofu – Tomato Soup

Two servings

Cook for 30-40 minutes:
> **½ cup uncooked brown rice**
> **1½ cups water**

In a separate saucepan, simmer for 10 minutes:
> **4 medium tomatoes, chopped**
> **½ cup onion, chopped**
> **½ tsp. basil**
> **½ tsp. pepper**
> **½ tsp. kelp**

Puree vegetables in blender and set aside.

In a large pot, stir together:
> **2 Tbsps. whole wheat flour**
> **¼ cup low-fat soymilk powder**
> **2 cups low-fat soymilk**

Add and heat:
> **8 oz. reduced-fat tofu, diced**
> **the cooked rice**
> **the tomato puree**

Simmer, stirring every few minutes.

Stir in:
> **1 Tbsp. parsley or chives**

Per serving: Calories: 419, 1½ meats, 2 breads, 1 milk, 2 vegetables
Protein: 14 gm., Fat: 3 gm., Carbohydrates: 73 gm., Percentage of calories from fat: 7%

Tofu Vegetable Soup

One serving

Cook for 15 minutes:

> **2 Tbsps. uncooked brown rice**
> **2 cups water**

Add and simmer 10-15 minutes longer:

> **¾ cup carrots, sliced**
> **1 small potato, diced**
> **¼ cup fresh or frozen peas**
> **½ cup celery, sliced**
> **½ cup onions, chopped**
> **tarragon, bay leaf, basil, celery seed to taste**

Stir in:

> **8 oz. firm low-fat tofu, cut into bite-sized pieces**

Per serving: Calories: 405, 3 meats, 2 breads, 2 vegetables
Protein: 11 gm., Fat: 1 gm., Carbohydrates: 69 gm., Percentage of calories from fat: 3%

Main Dishes

✛

Baked Tofu

Three servings

Have ready:
> **1 lb. low-fat tofu, sliced**

Marinate tofu for 1 hour in:
> **3 Tbsps. tamari**
> **2 Tbsps. onion, finely chopped**
> **1 Tbsp. Herb Mix (page 138)**
> **1 Tbsp. canola oil**

Bake on cookie sheet for 20 minutes at 375°F. Turn over after 10 minutes, and sprinkle with:
> **fresh chives**

Per serving: Calories: 131, 1 meat, 1 fat
> *Protein: 5 gm., Fat: 5 gm., Carbohydrates: 2 gm. Percentage of calories from fat: 34%*

Cashew-Carrot Parmesan

Three servings

Simmer for 15 minutes:
>**½ cup uncooked millet**
>**1½ cups water**
>**1 tsp. oregano**

In a separate medium saucepan, simmer for 5 minutes:
>**½ cup diced carrots**
>**½ cup onion, chopped**
>**½ cup water**
>**½ tsp. oregano**
>**1 tsp. vegetable broth powder**

Drain cooking water from the vegetables into the millet, and keep on low heat until the water is absorbed.

Preheat oven to 350°F.

Mix into vegetables:
>**½ cup cashews, broken**

Add:
>**the cooked millet**
>**9 oz. tofu, sliced ½" thick**

Place in an ungreased, 1-quart casserole dish.

Sprinkle with:
>**3 Tbsps. soy Parmesan**

Bake for 10-15 minutes.

Per serving: Calories: 423, 3 meats, 1½ breads, 1 vegetable, 1 fat
    Protein: 16 gm., Fat: 16 gm., Carbohydrates: 54 gm., Percentage of calories from fat: 33%

Cashew Loaf

Six servings

This loaf reminds me of a bread stuffing, but with the protein built right in.
For non-stick pan, eliminate oil, eliminate ½ fat.

Have ready:

6 slices whole wheat bread, crumbled
3 cups cashews, ground

Preheat oven to 350°F.

Mix above ingredients together in order given with:

3 Tbsps. nutritional yeast
3 Tbsps. parsley, chopped
½ tsp. sage
½ tsp. basil
½ tsp. marjoram
½ tsp. oregano
2 cups onion, chopped
1 cup low-fat soymilk

Place in a 9" x 13" casserole which has been greased with:

1 tsp. oil

Bake for 35-40 minutes.

Per serving: Calories: 551, 3 meats, 2 breads, 2 fat
*   Protein: 51 gm., Fat: 34 gm., Carbohydrates: 43 gm., Percentage of calories from fat: 57%*

Far East Fried Rice

Two servings

Cut into strips or dice:
8 oz. tofu or 8 oz. tempeh (steamed for 10 minutes and cooled)

Simmer for 45 minutes until liquid is absorbed:
½ cup brown rice
1½ cups water

Heat in wok or skillet:
1 Tbsp. oil

Add and brown lightly:
2 Tbsps. sesame seeds

Add and brown:
the tofu or tempeh

Stir in:
¼ cup onions, sliced
½ cup celery, sliced
4 spinach leaves, shredded

Sauté a few minutes, then add:
the cooked rice

Mix all ingredients together, and add:
4 tsps. tamari

Sprinkle on top to serve:
¼ cup green onions, chopped

Per serving: Calories: 329, 2 meats, 1 bread, 2 fats
Protein: 9 gm., Fat: 12 gm., Carbohydrates: 38 gm., Percentage of calories from fat: 33%

Grainburgers

Makes 8 burgers

Mix:

> **2 cups cooked brown rice**
> **⅓ cup cornmeal**
> **⅓ cup whole wheat flour**
> **⅓ cup oatmeal**
> **2 Tbsps. dried parsley**
> **1 tsp. tumeric**
> **1 tsp. garlic powder**
> **½ tsp. salt**

Simmer in ½ cup water for 10 minutes:

> **⅓ cup celery, chopped**
> **⅓ cup onion, chopped**

Mix celery and onion into dry ingredients along with:

> **½ cup low-fat tofu, mashed**

Form eight patties and brown each side in on a non-stick skillet:

Per burger: Calories: 75, ½ bread, ½ meat
   Protein: 3 gm., Fat: 0 gm., Carbohydrates: 14 gm., Percentage of calories from fat: 10%

Mediterranean Broccoli and Rice

Four servings

Crumble into a small pan and toast:

2 slices whole wheat bread
1 tsp. oil

Set aside.

Simmer together over low heat for 45 minutes:

1 cup uncooked brown rice
3 cups water
¼ tsp. each pepper, bay, basil, and tarragon
½ tsp. oregano
½ tsp. kelp
½ cup onion, chopped

Mix in:

10.5 oz. low-fat tofu, mashed
2 Tbsps. nutritional yeast
1 (10 oz.) package frozen chopped broccoli, cooked

Place mixture in an ungreased 8" x 8" casserole dish, and top with:

4 oz. soy cheese, grated
the toasted bread crumbs

Heat in the oven for a few minutes to melt cheese.

Per serving: Calories: 328, 3 meats, 2 breads
   Protein: 16 gm., Fat: 10 gm., Carbohydrates: 43 gm., Percentage of calories from fat: 28%

Millet with Peas and Sesame

Two servings

Simmer over low heat until liquid is absorbed:

½ cup uncooked millet
2 cups water
½ cup onion, chopped
1 tsp. salt free vegetable bouillon

Toast in a dry skillet for a few minutes to lightly brown:

¼ cup sesame seeds

Mix into the cooked millet:

1 cup cooked fresh or blanched frozen peas
the toasted sesame seeds

Per serving: Calories: 391, 2 meats, 2 breads, 1 fat, 1 vegetable
Protein: 13 gm., Fat: 10 gm., Carbohydrates: 60 gm., Percentage of calories from fat: 24%

Millet with Tofu & Mushrooms

Four servings

Cook together for 20 minutes:

4 cups water
1 cup uncooked millet
1 clove garlic, minced
½ cup scallions, chopped
2 Tbsps. parsley, minced

Preheat over to 350°F.

Sauté together:

1 tsp. canola oil
1 cup mushrooms, chopped

Add to mushrooms:

1 (10.5 oz.) package low-fat tofu, cubed

Combine millet with mushrooms and tofu. Spoon into a lightly oiled 8" x 8" baking dish. Bake, covered for 20-25 minutes.

Per serving: Calories: 351, 2 meats, 1 bread, ½ fat,
    Protein: 14 gm., Fat: 5 gm., Carbohydrates: 62 gm., Percentage of calories from fat: 13%

Oriental Tofu

Two servings

Simmer for 5 minutes:

1 cup mushrooms, sliced or halved
½ cup onions, sliced
½ cup water

Add and cook about 35 minutes more until rice is tender:

⅓ cup uncooked brown rice
⅓ cup water
1 tsp. tamari

Add and cook another 5 minutes:
6 oz. firm tofu, diced

Per serving: Calories: 204, 1½ meat, 1 bread, 1 vegetable
Protein: 10 gm., Fat: 4 gm., Carbohydrates: 31 gm., Percentage of calories from fat: 18%

Quinoa Pilaf

Four servings

Add:
>   **1 cup uncooked quinoa**

To:
>   **2 cups boiling water**

Cover and cook for 15 minutes. Turn off heat and leave grain covered for 10 minutes.

Sauté:
>   **1 cup onions, chopped**
>   **2 cloves garlic, minced**
>   **1 Tbsp. olive oil**

Fluff quinoa with fork, add onions and garlic. Salt to taste if desired.

Per serving: Calories: 197, 1 bread, 1 fat, 1 vegetable
*   Protein: 7 gm., Fat: 6 gm., Carbohydrates: 30 gm., Percentage of calories from fat: 25%*

Tofu-Cauliflower Curry

Two servings

Sauté all ingredients together until cauliflower is crispy but tender:
>   **1 Tbsp. canola oil**
>   **10.5 oz. low-fat tofu, diced**
>   **2 cups cauliflower, chopped**
>   **½ cup onion, chopped**
>   **½ tsp. salt**
>   **¼ tsp. pepper**
>   **1 tsp. curry**

Per serving: Calories: 185, 1½ meats, 1 vegetable, 1 fat
*   Protein: 6 gm., Fat: 8 gm., Carbohydrates: 8 gm. Percentage of calories from fat: 35%*

Sesame Tofu

Six slices

Use a non-stick pan.

Mix together in a small bowl:
> **1 Tbsp. tamari**
> **2 Tbsps. water**

In another bowl, combine:
> **¼ cup sesame seed**
> **¼ cup wheat germ**

Slice into 6 slices:
> **12 oz. reduced-fat tofu**

Dip each slice into the tamari then into the dry mixture.

Fry 3 slices at a time in:
> **a drop of oil**

Serve with rice or another grain or in a sandwich with lettuce and tomato.

Per slice: Calories: 78, 1 meat
> *Protein: 4 gm., Fat: 3 gm., Carbohydrates: 4 gm., Percentage of calories from fat: 38%*

Soft Tacos

Makes 8 tacos

Preheat oven to 350°F.

2 cups pinto beans, cooked
8 corn tortillas

Heat beans. Place 2 Tbsps. in each tortilla, fold, and place upright in a baking dish.

In a small saucepan, combine and cook slowly until thick:

¼ cup salsa
2 Tbsps. soy yogurt
1 Tbsp. flour

Pour sauce over tortillas and heat in oven for 10 minutes.

Each taco: Calories: 133, 1 bread, 1 meat
Protein: 5 gm., Fat: 1 gm., Carbohydrates: 25 gm. Percentage of calories from fat: 9%

Stir-Fry Vegetables with Tofu

Two servings

Heat in skillet:

2 tsps. oil

Add:

8 oz. low-fat tofu, cubed
2 cups vegetables, chopped (celery, peppers, onion, peas, carrots, broccoli)
2 Tbsps. tamari

Cook over medium-high heat, stirring to prevent sticking.

Per serving: Calories: 194, 1 meat, 2 vegetables, 1 fat
Protein: 11 gm., Fat: 9 gm., Carbohydrates: 13 gm. Percentage of calories from fat: 23%

Soybean-Mushroom Pilaf

Four servings

Have ready and warmed:

3 cups cooked rice
1½ cups cooked soybeans

Simmer until greens are tender:

2 cups mushrooms, chopped
¼ cup onion, chopped
2 Tbsps. parsley
1 cup kale or spinach, chopped
2 tsps. oil
¼ cup water

Stir in rice and soybeans.

Per serving: Calories: 320, 2 meats, 2 breads, 1 vegetable
Protein: 14 gm., Fat: 8 gm., Carbohydrates: 47 gm., Percentage of calories from fat: 23%

Soyburgers

Three servings

Mash:
>**1 cup cooked soybeans**

Mix with:
>**2 Tbsps. nutritional yeast**
>**1 cup oatmeal**
>**1 Tbsp. tamari**

Preheat oven to 350°F.

Sauté:
>**¼ cup onion, chopped**
>**1 clove garlic, minced**
>**½ tsp. oregano**
>**½ tsp. basil**
>**1 Tbsp. oil**

Add to the beans. Mix well and form 6 flat patties. Bake on ungreased cookie sheet for 10 minutes.

Turn and top with:
>**¼ cup tomato sauce**

Bake 10-15 minutes more.

Per serving of 2 patties: Calories: 218, 2 meats, 1 bread, 1 fat
Protein: 16 gm., Fat: 10 gm., Carbohydrates: 29 gm., Percentage of calories from fat: 32%

Tempeh with Mushroom Stuffing

One serving

Here is a quick and delicious tempeh recipe.

Preheat oven to 350°F.

Simmer together:
> **2 Tbsps. tomato sauce**
> **½ cup mushrooms, chopped**
> **¼ cup onions, chopped**
> **1 clove garlic, minced**
> **dash black pepper**
> **2 Tbsps. water**

Remove from heat and mix in until hot:
> **2 slices whole wheat bread, crumbled**
> **3 Tbsps. soy Parmesan cheese**

Lay in a dish and cover with mixture:
> **4 oz. piece of tempeh, sliced in half and steamed for**
> **10 minutes**

Bake covered for 15 minutes.

Per serving: Calories: 494, 4 meats, 2 breads, 2 vegetables
> *Protein: 35 gm., Fat: 13 gm., Carbohydrates: 59 gm., Percentage of calories from fat: 23%*

Tofu Lasagne

Two servings

Cook in boiling water until tender:
> **4 oz. whole wheat or enriched lasagne noodles**

Drain noodles and set aside.

Mix:
> **½ cup tomato sauce**
> **½ cup steamed broccoli, finely chopped**

Preheat oven to 350°F.

In a 9" x 5" loaf pan layer half the noodles with:
> **8 oz. firm tofu, crumbled**
> **2 oz. soy mozzarella cheese, grated**

Top with the rest of the noodles, tomato sauce mixture and:
> **3 Tbsps. soy Parmesan cheese**

Bake until hot, about 10 minutes.

Per serving: Calories: 297, 2 meats, 1 bread
> *Protein: 19 gm., Fat: 13 gm., Carbohydrates: 24 gm., Percentage of calories from fat: 40%*

Tofu–Mushroom Pot Pies

Four servings

Crust

Mix together with a fork:
>   1¼ cups whole wheat pastry flour
>   ¼ cup wheat germ
>   3 Tbsps. oil
>   2-3 Tbsps. water

Break into 4 pieces, roll out each piece, and place in 4 oven proof dishes.

Filling

Simmer for 10 minutes:
>   2 cups mushrooms, chopped
>   1 cup celery, chopped with leaves
>   ½ cup onion, chopped
>   1 Tbsp. salt-free bouillon powder
>   ½ cup water

Preheat oven to 350°F.

Stir in:
>   12 oz. tofu, diced

Divide filling into 4 oven proof dishes. Bake for 30 minutes.

Per serving: Calories: 327, 2 meats, 2 breads, 1 fat
*   Protein: 14 gm., Fat: 14 gm., Carbohydrates: 34 gm., Percentage of calories from fat: 39%*

Tofu-Mushroom Quiche

Six servings

This recipe is shown on the front cover.

Prepare crust:

1 cup unbleached white flour
3 Tbsps. canola oil
¼ cup water
pinch of salt

Mix ingredients together. Roll out on floured surface, and place into a 9" pie pan.

Preheat oven to 350°F.

Prepare filling:

12 mushrooms, chopped
1 medium red bell pepper, chopped
1 cup broccoli florets, chopped
¼ tsp. black pepper
¼ tsp. basil
¼ tsp. thyme
¼ tsp. bay leaves, ground
1 Tbsp. spicy mustard
12 oz. low-fat tofu, blended

Sauté vegetables and spices in a small amount of water until vegetables are crisp-tender. Blend tofu until smooth and mix with vegetables. Spoon into pie crust and bake for 20-25 minutes.

Garnish top with:

toasted sesame seeds, cashews, and green onions (optional)

Per serving: Calories: 171, 1 meat, 1 fat, 1 bread,
*   Protein: 4 gm., Fat: 7 gm., Carbohydrates: 17 gm., Percentage of calories from fat: 39%*

Tofu-Oatmeal Casserole

Four servings

Preheat oven to 350°F.

Bring to a boil and simmer for 10 minutes:

2 cups water
½ cup onion, chopped
2 cups mixture of celery, carrots, and mushrooms, chopped
1 tsp. garlic powder
2 tsps. dried parsley
1 tsp. oregano
½ tsp. savory

Add:

2 cups oatmeal
1 Tbsp. nutritional yeast
1 lb. low-fat tofu, mashed

Press into an oiled baking dish. Bake for 20 minutes. During last 5 minutes of baking, sprinkle on top:

3 Tbsps. sunflower seeds

Per serving: Calories: 236, 1 meat, 1 bread, 1 vegetable
Protein: 10 gm., Fat: 5 gm., Carbohydrates: 28 gm. Percentage of calories from fat: 21%

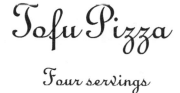

Tofu Pizza

Four servings

CRUST

Preheat oven to 350°F.

Dissolve together:
½ cup warm water
1 Tbsp. yeast

Mix in:
1 cup whole wheat flour
⅓ cup oatmeal

Beat the mixture well. Roll out dough, place in a lightly oiled and floured pie plate and bake for 15 minutes.

TOPPING

Mix together:
1 (10.5 oz.) package low-fat tofu, diced
⅓ cup tomato sauce
¼ cup soy Parmesan cheese

When crust is ready, pour on tofu mixture, and top with:
4 oz. soy mozzarella, grated

You can also add a few sliced green peppers, onions, or mushrooms along with the cheese. Bake for 10-15 minutes more at 350°F until crust is done and cheese is melted.

Per serving: Calories: 276, 2 meats, 2 breads, 1 vegetable
    Protein: 17 gm., Fat: 9 gm., Carbohydrates: 30 gm., Percentage of calories from fat: 32%

Tofu Shepherd's Pie

Four servings

Preheat oven to 350°F.
> **6 medium potatoes, mashed**

Wash and peel potatoes. Steam for about 15 minutes or until soft. Place in a bowl and mash potatoes with a little water or soy milk. Line the bottom of a lightly oiled pie pan with the mashed potatoes. Put the following mixture on top of the potatoes:
> **1 lb. low-fat tofu, mashed**
> **2 tsps. herb mix**
> **1 cup onions, chopped**
> **1 cup celery, chopped**
> **1 cup carrots, chopped**

Sprinkle on top:
> **1 slice whole wheat bread, crumbled**
> **fresh parsley, chopped**

Bake for 15 minutes

Per serving: Calories: 280, 1½ meats, 1½ breads, 2 vegetables, ½ fat
*   Protein: 7 gm., Fat: 1 gm., Carbohydrates: 51 gm., Percentage of calories from fat: 3%*

TVP® Meatless Loaf

Four servings

Preheat oven to 350°F.

Mix and set aside for 15 minutes:

1½ cups TVP® granules
1 tsp. basil
½ garlic powder
½ oregano
¼ cup fresh parsley, chopped
¼ tsp. salt
1 cup whole wheat bread crumbs
1½ cups boiling water
¼ cup tomato sauce

Sauté onion in olive oil, and add to mixture:

½ cup onion, chopped
1 Tbsp. olive oil

Bake in a non-stick pan for 20 minutes.

Per serving: Calories: 157, 1 meat, 1 bread, ½ fat
Protein: 16 gm., Fat: 4 gm., Carbohydrates: 14 gm. Percentage of calories from fat: 22%

Vegetables

✛

Broccoli-Mushroom Casserole

Four servings

Preheat oven to 350°F.

Bring water to a boil. Simmer broccoli, mushrooms, onion, and garlic for 3 minutes:

> **1 cup water**
> **2 cups broccoli, chopped**
> **2 cups mushrooms, chopped**
> **½ cup onion, chopped**
> **2 cloves garlic, minced**

Add:

> **2 cups oatmeal**
> **¼ cup sesame seeds**
> **8 oz. low-fat tofu, mashed**

Mix together well. Put into an oiled baking dish, and bake for 15 minutes. Top with:

> **½ cup tomato sauce**

Bake 5 minutes more and serve.

Per serving: Calories: 287, 2 meats, 1 bread, 2 vegetables
Protein: 12 gm., Fat: 8 gm., Carbohydrates: 37 gm. Percentage of calories from fat: 23%

Corn-Crunchy Garbanzos

Two servings

Cook over low heat for thirty minutes:

⅓ cup uncooked brown rice
1 cup water
¼ tsp. sage
¼ tsp. thyme
½ tsp. rosemary
1 clove garlic, chopped
2 Tbsps. parsley
½ cup onion, chopped

Stir in and heat:

½ cup frozen corn
1 cup cooked garbanzo beans

For topping, heat in pan:

3 Tbsps. sesame seeds
¼ cup wheat germ
2 tsps. oil

Mix until seeds and wheat germ are coated with oil. Sprinkle topping over the beans and rice.

Per serving: Calories: 432, 3 meat, 1 bread, 2½ fat
  Protein: 15 gm., Fat: 14 gm., Carbohydrates: 60 gm., Percentage of calories from fat: 28%

Elbow Macaroni with Cashew "Cheese"

Two servings

This really does taste similar to macaroni and cheese, but without the animal fat, and the recipe can easily be doubled to serve four.

Cook in boiling water (salted if not on a salt-free diet):
   2 cups whole wheat or enriched elbow macaroni

Drain and set aside.

Sauce:

Blend to a fine powder in the blender:
   ½ cup cashews

Add and blend again:
   ½ pepper, chopped
   ½ onion, chopped
   2 Tbsps. nutritional yeast
   2 Tbsps. lemon juice
   1 clove garlic, minced
   1½ cups water

Topping:

Mix together in a small saucepan:
   ¼ cup mixture of bran and wheat germ
   1 Tbsp. nutritional yeast
   1 tsp. oil
   1 Tbsp. parsley

Sauté until hot, but not browned. Preheat oven to 350°F. Place sauce in a pan with the cooked macaroni. Stir and heat until thick. Pour into an 8" x 8" ungreased casserole dish, and bake for 10 minutes. Top with topping and return to oven for 5 more minutes.

Per serving: Calories: 509, 3 meats, 2 breads, 2½ fats
   Protein: 19 gm., Fat: 21 gm., Carbohydrates: 60 gm., Percentage of calories from fat: 36%

Mushroom Supper Cake

Two servings

This is a very filling supper, served with a salad and vegetables.

Simmer in a covered frying pan for 10 minutes:

1 cup mushrooms, chopped
½ cup peppers & onions, chopped
2 cloves garlic, minced
1 Tbsp. vegetable broth powder
½ cup water

Remove from heat and mix in:

4 slices whole wheat bread, crumbled

Allow bread to soak up flavors for 10 minutes.

Preheat oven to 350°F.

Beat in:

2 Tbsps. soy Parmesan
¾ cup low-fat tofu, crumbled

Bake for 15 minutes in a lightly oiled shallow dish.

Sprinkle on:

1 Tbsp. soy Parmesan

Return to the oven and bake 5 more minutes.

Per serving: Calories: 248, 1 meat, 2 breads, ½ fat, 1 vegetable
    Protein: 18 gm., Fat: 7 gm., Carbohydrates: 26 gm., Percentage of calories from fat: 26%

Non-Dairy Scalloped Potatoes

Six servings

Preheat oven to 350°F.

Sauté together:
>   1 tsp. olive oil
>   1 large onion, sliced
>   4 cloves garlic, minced

Add:
>   1½ cups water
>   ¼ cup tahini
>   2 Tbsps. whole wheat flour
>   1 tsp. salt (optional)

Stir until thick.

Steam 15 minutes or until soft:
>   6-7 medium potatoes, sliced

Layer potatoes in a casserole dish, and pour onion/tahini mixture over top. Sprinkle with:
>   2 Tbsps. parsley

Cook uncovered for 10-15 minutes.

Per serving: Calories: 226, 2 fats, 1 meat, 1 bread
*   Protein: 4 gm., Fats: 5 gm., Carbohydrates: 39 gm. Percentage of calories from fat: 23%*

Oven Eggplant

Two servings

Cook in boiling water, covered, for 5 minutes:
1 medium eggplant

Drain and cut in two, lengthwise. Scoop out the insides, leaving a half- inch shell.

Mash eggplant with:
½ cup tofu, mashed
2 Tbsps. onion, chopped
1 tsp. bay leaves, ground
1 tsp. basil
1 tsp. oregano
2 Tbsps. tomato sauce

Preheat oven to 350°F.

Stuff eggplant halves, place in casserole, and bake covered for 15 minutes. Add a little water to the bottom of the dish to keep eggplant moist.

Top with:
2 Tbsps. wheat germ
2 Tbsps. soy Parmesan (optional)

Bake 5 more minutes, uncovered.

Per serving: Calories: 240, 2 meats, ½ bread, 2 vegetables
Protein: 11 gm., Fat: 10 gm., Carbohydrates: 26 gm., Percentage of calories from fat: 36%

Sesame Potatoes

Four servings

Use a non-stick pan.

Steam until almost done:

2 cups diced potatoes (with skins)
1 cup fresh peas (If 1 cup frozen peas are substituted, they do not need to be cooked)

Preheat oven to 350°F.

Mix in:

2 Tbsps. onion, chopped
1 Tbsp. parsley, chopped
1 cup low-fat tofu, crumbled
2 Tbsps. sesame seed

Place in a lightly oiled 8" x 8" casserole, and top with:

3 Tbsps. soy Parmesan
1 Tbsp. sesame seed

Bake uncovered for 30 minutes.

Per serving: Calories: 214, 1½ meats, 1½ breads, 1 fat
Protein: 15 gm., Fat: 5 gm., Carbohydrates: 27 gm., Percentage of calories from fat: 24%

Sweet Potato Rice

Two servings

Cook over low heat for 40 minutes:

⅔ cup uncooked rice
2 cups water

Stir in and heat thoroughly:

2 Tbsps. fresh parsley, chopped
¼ tsp. sage
½ cup cooked sweet potato, mashed
¼ tsp. pepper
¼ tsp. wheat germ
1 Tbsp. nutritional yeast

Serve warm or cold with:

4 oz. soy yogurt

Per serving: Calories: 340, 2 meats, 2 breads, 1 fat
Protein: 10 gm., Fat: 3 gm., Carbohydrates: 65 gm., Percentage of calories from fat: 7%

Sweet Potatoes and Broccoli

One serving

Cook in covered sauce pan until almost done:
1 medium sweet potato or yam, diced (1 cup)
½ cup water

Add and cook until tender:
1 cup fresh broccoli, chopped
additional water to cook, if necessary

Toss in with vegetables until hot:
½ cup low-fat tofu, crumbled
1 Tbsp. sesame seeds

Per Serving: Calories: 285, 2 meats, ½ bread, 1 fat, 2 vegetables
Protein: 13 gm., Fat: 7 gm., Carbohydrates: 46 gm., Percentage of calories from fat: 15%

Beans

It's a good idea to cook up some beans whenever you have the time, so you will have them for preparing a quick meal. Cooked beans will last about a week in the refrigerator, or can be frozen in measured portions. Many of the recipes in this section are also good to take along cold for lunch.

Falafel

Four servings

Preheat oven to 350°F.

Grind in a food processor or blender:

3 cups cooked garbanzo beans
1 Tbsp. lemon juice
½ cup onion, chopped

Remove and mix with:

2 Tbsps. whole wheat pastry flour
¼ cup wheat germ
¼ cup parsley
¼ cup sesame seed
¼ tsp. pepper
¼ tsp. garlic powder

Form into 20 falafel balls.

Heat in a large baking dish in the oven:

2 Tbsps. oil

Place falafel in the dish, and bake 15 minutes, stirring occasionally.

Per serving of 5 falafels: Calories: 552, 3½ meats, 2 breads, 3 fats
   Protein: 21 gm., Fat: 14 gm., Carbohydrates: 82 gm., Percentage of calories from fat: 23%

Garbanzo – Rice Casserole

Four servings

Simmer for 40 minutes:

> **1 cup brown rice**
> **3 cups water**
> **1 tsp. basil**
> **¼ cup onion, chopped**
> **¼ cup green pepper, chopped**

Preheat oven to 350°F.

Mix in:

> **2 cups cooked garbanzo beans**
> **2 Tbsps. tahini**

Grease an 8" x 8" casserole dish with:

> **1 tsp. oil**

Place mixture in dish and bake for 10 minutes.

Top with:

> **⅓ cup soy cheese, grated (optional)**

Return to oven and bake for 10 more minutes.

Per serving: Calories: 340, 2 meats, 2 breads, 1½ fats
   Protein: 11 gm., Fat: 7 gm., Carbohydrates: 57 gm., Percentage of calories from fat: 18%

Hearty Beans and Rice Supper

Four servings

Simmer over low heat for 35 minutes:

⅔ cup rice
1½ cups water
1 cup celery, chopped
½ cup onion, chopped
½ cup green pepper, chopped
½ tsp. bay leaves, ground
½ tsp. basil
½ tsp. oregano

Mix in and cook 10 minutes:

2 cups cooked pinto beans
1 cup fresh or frozen corn
2 fresh tomatoes, chopped
1 tsp. olive oil

Per serving: Calories: 187, 1 meat, 1 bread, 1 vegetable
Protein: 8 gm., Fat: 1 gm., Carbohydrates: 35 gm., Percentage of calories from fat: 7%

Patty's Garbanzo Patties

Four servings

Simmer in 1 cup water for 10 minutes:
>   **1 clove garlic, crushed**
>   **1 cup mushrooms, chopped**

Stir in and then blend:
>   **1 cup cooked garbanzo beans**
>   **¼ cup tomato sauce**
>   **½ cup onion, chopped**

Mix ground beans with:
>   **1 cup whole cooked garbanzo beans**
>   **4 slices whole wheat bread, crumbled**
>   **⅓ cup sesame seeds**
>   **⅓ cup oatmeal**
>   **⅓ cup rolled wheat or oats**
>   **1 Tbsp. nutritional yeast**
>   **1 Tbsp. herb mix (page 138)**

Set aside for twelve minutes. Form twelve patties and cook on non-stick pan.

Per serving (3 patties): Calories: 340, 2 meats, 2 breads, 1 fat
Protein: 15 gm., Fat: 9 gm., Carbohydrates: 48 gm., Percentage of calories from fat: 23%

Pinto Bean Loaf

Four servings

*This loaf is good topped with soy yogurt. I use about ½ cup soy yogurt for each serving.
Add ½ milk exchange.*

Have ready:
2 slices whole wheat bread, crumbled
2 cups cooked pinto beans
½ cup peanuts, ground
½ cup celery, chopped
½ cup onion, chopped

Preheat oven to 350°F.

Mix above ingredients together with:
⅔ cup oatmeal
¾ cup water

Place mixture in a small loaf pan or an 8" x 8" casserole which has been greased with:
1 tsp. oil

Bake covered for 20-25 minutes.

Per serving: Calories: 351, 3 meats, 1 bread, 1 fat
Protein: 14 gm., Fat: 13 gm., Carbohydrates: 42 gm., Percentage of Calories from fat: 42%

Pintos and Pasta

One serving

This recipe can easily be doubled or quadrupled.

Boil until tender (about 10 minutes):
>   **½ cup whole wheat or enriched elbow macaroni**
>   **1 cup water**

Sauté until tender:
>   **1 Tbsp. onion, chopped**
>   **1 tsp. olive oil**

Add and simmer:
>   **1 Tbsp. tomato sauce**
>   **½ cup pinto beans, cooked**
>   **2 Tbsps. sesame seeds**

Stir in macaroni.

Per serving: Calories: 518, 3 meats, 2 breads, 1 fat
*   Protein: 24 gm., Fat: 16 gm., Carbohydrates: 69 gm., Percentage of calories from fat: 27%*

Pintos with Cornbread Topping

Four servings

You can try reversing this and using the topping on the bottom and the beans on top.
Either way it's great!

Simmer over medium heat for 10 minutes:

3 cups cooked pinto beans
⅓ cup tomato sauce
⅓ cup onion, chopped
⅓ cup green pepper, chopped

Preheat oven to 400°F.

For topping, mix in a small bowl:

4 tsps. canola oil
1 cup cornmeal
1 cup low-fat soymilk
1 tsp. chili powder (optional)

Put beans in an 8" x 8" dish, then pour cornmeal mixture on top, and bake for 15-20 minutes, uncovered.

Per serving: Calories: 374, 2½ meats, 2 breads, 1 fat
    Protein: 13 gm., Fat: 6 gm., Carbohydrates: 66 gm., Percentage of calories from fat: 14%

Walnut-Lentil Loaf

Four servings

Curry powder to taste can be used in place of thyme, basil, and oregano.

Have ready:

1 slice whole wheat bread, crumbled
2 cups cooked lentils

Blend:

½ cup walnuts
½ cup onions
½ cup water

Preheat oven to 350°F.

Mix together above ingredients in order given with:

½ cup wheat germ
2 Tbsps. sesame seeds
½ tsp. thyme
¼ tsp. basil
¼ tsp. oregano
2 Tbsps. nutritional yeast
½ cup water
1 Tbsp. tomato sauce

Place mixture in a small loaf or in a 8" x 8" dish which has been greased with:

1 tsp. oil

Bake for 35-40 minutes.

Per serving: Calories: 341, 3 meats, 1 bread, 2 fats
  Protein: 17 gm., Fat: 14 gm., Carbohydrates: 36 gm., Percentage of calories from fat: 35%

Nutritional Yeast Sauce

You can use this sauce with pasta, vegetables, or grains.

Makes about 1½ cups

2 tsp. soy margarine
1 cup water
½ cup nutritional yeast
¼ cup whole wheat flour
¼ tsp salt (optional)
⅓ cup soy Parmesan

Melt soy margarine in a pan, and mix in the dry ingredients. Over medium heat, add water slowly, stirring constantly until mixture begins to thicken.

Per tablespoon: Calories 22
Protein: 2 gm., Fat: 0 gm., Carbohydrates: 2 gm., Percentage of calories from fat: 16%

White Pasta Sauce

Makes 2 cups

This sauce can be used over potatoes, pasta, or any grain.

2 tsp. soy margarine
⅓ cup whole wheat flour
⅓ cup soy Parmesan
2 Tbsp. Herb Mix (page 138)
2 cups low-fat soymilk

Melt margarine in a pan, and mix in flour, Parmesan, and herbs. Slowly add soymilk over medium heat, and stir until thick.

Per tablespoon.: Calories 17, (If you use a half cup per serving add 1 fat)
Protein: 1 gm., Fat: 0 gm., Carbohydrates: 2 gm., Percentage of Calories from fat: 23%

Snacks

If you can make your snacks interesting and different, you will be less tempted to eat something you shouldn't, like potato chips or packaged cookies. Don't think of it as something you just want to get over with because you have to eat at a certain time. Take your time and make it enjoyable!

Apple-Oat Drop Cookies

Makes 20 cookies

Mash together with a fork:

      1½ cups oatmeal
      1 Tbsp. whole wheat flour
      2 medium apples, grated
      1 Tbsp. oil
      ½ tsp. vanilla
      ¼ cup water

Mix in:

      ½ cup raisins
      ¼ cup finely chopped walnuts

Let the mixture soak together in the bowl for 15 minutes. Preheat oven to 350°F. Drop by tablespoons onto an ungreased baking sheet. Bake for 10-12 minutes.

Per cookie: Calories 61, ½ bread, 1 fat
   Protein: 1 gm., Fat: 2 gm., Carbohydrates: 9 gm., Percentage of Calories from fat: 30%

Banana Split

One serving

Split in half lengthwise:
1 banana

Top in order given with:
½ cup soy yogurt
6 walnuts, chopped
2 Tbsps. wheat germ

Per serving: Calories: 333, 2 fruits, 1 fat, ½ milk, 1 bread; or 2 fruits, 1 fat, 1 milk
Protein: 13 gm., Fat: 12 gm., Carbohydrates: 41 gm., Percentage of calories from fat: 33%

Northern Fruit Salad

Four servings

Toss together:
2 medium apples, diced
2 medium pears, diced
10 cherries, pitted
10 grapes
2 tsps. lemon juice

Per serving: Calories: 107, 2 fruits
Protein: 1 gm., Fat: 0 gm., Carbohydrates: 25 gm., Percentage of calories from fat: 2%

Popcorn

One serving

This is a good snack for a person with diabetes because of the large, satisfying quantity that is allowed for 1 bread. Without butter or salt, it is low in calories and provides good roughage and some trace minerals. Here are some other ingredients which can be added to popcorn to create new snack ideas. (⅓ cup unpopped popcorn will equal 3 cups popped for 90 calories and 1 bread exchange)

To three cups of popcorn:

Mix in:

2 Tbsps. soy Parmesan
1 Tbsp. peanuts

Calories: 213, 1 bread, 2 fats, ½ milk
   Protein: 11 gm., Fat: 7 gm., Carbohydrates: 25 gm., Percentage of calories from fat: 30%

This is really a unique and tasty combination.

Sprinkle on:
1 Tbsp. nutritional yeast

Calories: 92, 1 bread
   Protein: 6 gm., Fat: 1 gm., Carbohydrates: 20 gm., Percentage of calories from fat: 8%

Quick Rice Pudding

Two servings

Preheat oven to 350°F.

Mix together in order given:
- **1 cup cooked brown rice**
- **1 cup low-fat soymilk**
- **1½ Tbsps. raisins**

Divide into 2 small serving dishes, and sprinkle with:
- **1 tsp. nutmeg**

Bake 15 minutes, then refrigerate

Per serving: Calories: 158, 1 bread, 1 fruit, 1 milk
   Protein: 4 gm., Fat: 1 gm., Carbohydrates: 34 gm., Percentage of calories from fat: 6%

Tropical Fruit Salad

Four servings

Pictured on the cover.

Toss together:
- **4 fresh apricots or plums, pitted & cut up, or 1 cup grapes**
- **½ cup fresh, raspberries**
- **1 orange, peeled and cut into wedges**
- **1 cup fresh pineapple, diced**
- **1 banana, sliced**
- **2 Tbsps. unsweetened coconut**
- **2 tsps. lemon juice**

Per serving: Calories: 129, 2 fruits, ½ fat
   Protein: 2 gm., Fat: 4 gm., Carbohydrates: 20 gm., Percentage of calories from fat: 32%

The Winter Warmer

One serving

Preheat oven to 375°F.

Place in small casserole dish:
> **1 cup diced potatoes**

Add:
> **1 Tbsp water**
> **1 Tbsp cider vinegar**
> **¼ tsp each dill, oregano**
> **⅛ tsp pepper**

Stir to coat potatoes. Cover dish and bake for 20 minutes.

Per serving: Calories: 120, 1½ breads
   Protein: 2 gm., Fat: 0 gm., Carbohydrates: 28 gm., Percentage of calories from fat: 0%

Herb Mix

Makes 1½ cups

Combine ¼ cup each of these dried herbs:
> **oregano**
> **tarragon**
> **parsley**
> **garlic powder**
> **basil**
> **savory**

Place herbs in a glass jar, and stir. Add 1 or 2 tsp. salt if desired. Keep jar closed in a dark cool place.

Index

Ask your store to carry these books, or you may order directly from:

The Book Publishing Company
P.O. Box 99 Summertown, TN 38483

Or call: 1-800-695-2241
Please add $2.50 per book for shipping

Almost No Fat Cookbook 10.95
Almost No Fat Holiday Cookbook 12.95
Becoming Vegetarian 15.95
Burgers 'n Fries 'n Cinnamon Buns 6.95
Cookin' Healthy with One Foot Out the Door 8.95
Cooking with Gluten and Seitan 7.95
Ecological Cooking: Recipes to Save the Planet 10.95
Fabulous Beans 9.95
Foods that Cause You To Loose Weight 12.95
From The Global Kitchen 11.95
From A Traditional Greek Kitchen 11.95
Good Time Eatin' in Cajun Country 9.95
Holiday Diet Book 9.95
Indian Vegetarian Cooking at Your House 12.95
Instead of Chicken, Instead of Turkey 9.95
Judy Brown's Guide to Natural Foods Cooking 10.95
Kids Can Cook 9.95
New Farm Vegetarian Cookbook 8.95
Now & Zen Epicure 17.95
Olive Oil Cookery 11.95
Peaceful Cook 8.95
Physician's Slimming Guide 5.95
Power of Your Plate 12.95
Shiitake Way 7.95
Shoshoni Cookbook 12.95
Simply Heavenly 19.95
The Sprout Garden 9.95
Starting Over: Learning to Cook with Natural Foods 10.95
Tempeh Cookbook 10.95
Ten Talents (Vegetarian Cookbook) 18.95
Tofu Cookery 14.95
Tofu Quick and Easy 7.95
TVP® Cookbook 6.95
Uncheese Cookbook 11.95
Uprisings: The Whole Grain Bakers' Book 13.95